# SAQs for Dentistry

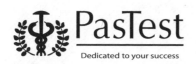
Dedicated to your success

# SAQs for Dentistry

**Kathleen F M Fan**
**PhD, BDS, MBBS, FDSRCS, FRCSEd, FRCS (OMFS)**
Specialist Registrar in Oral and Maxillofacial Surgery
London, Kent, Sussex and Surrey Rotation

**Judith Jones BDS, MSc, FDSRCS (Eng),**
**PhD, FDS, (OS), ILTM**
Lecturer/Honorary Consultant in Oral Surgery
King's College London Dental Institute
at Guy's, King's College and
St Thomas' Hospitals

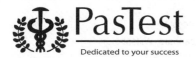

PasTest
Dedicated to your success

© 2007 PASTEST LTD
Egerton Court
Parkgate Estate
Knutsford
Cheshire
WA16 8DX
Telephone: 01565 752000

First Published 2007
ISBN: 1905635 1 68
ISBN: 978 1905635 160

A catalogue record for this book is available from the British Library.
The information contained within this book was obtained by the author from reliable
sources. However, while every effort has been made to ensure its accuracy, no
responsibility for loss, damage or injury occasioned to any person acting or refraining
from action as a result of information contained herein can be accepted by the
publishers or authors

---

**PasTest Revision Books and Intensive Courses**

PasTest has been established in the field of postgraduate medical education since
1972, providing revision books and intensive study courses for doctors preparing
for their professional examinations.

Books and courses are available for the following specialties:
**MRCGP, MRCP Parts 1 and 2, MRCPCH Parts 1 and 2, MRCPsych, MRCS,
MRCOG Parts 1 and 2, DRCOG, DCH, FRCA, PLAB Parts 1 and 2.**

For further details contact:
PasTest, Freepost, Knutsford, Cheshire WA16 7BR
**Tel: 01565 752000 Fax: 01565 650264**
**www.pastest.co.uk enquiries@pastest.co.uk**

---

Text prepared by Carnegie Book Production, Lancaster
Printed and bound by CPI Anthony Rowe, Chippenham, Wiltshire.

# Contents

# List of Contributors

Dr A W Barrett BDS MSc PhD FDS RCS (Ed & Eng) FRCPath
Consultant Oral Pathologist
Queen Victoria Hospital
East Grinstead

Julia Costello BDS MSc
Clinical Demonstrator Department of Periodontology
Guy's Hospital,
Kings College London

Richard Jones BDS MSc FDSRCS M. Orth.RCS
Specialist Orthodontic Practitioner
Total Orthodontic Ltd
Sussex

Dr Virginia J Kingsmill PhD BDS FDSRCS
Lecturer
Departement of Conservative Dentistry
Barts and The London Queen Mary School of Medicine and Dentistry

# Introduction

Methods of examining and assessing students have changed over recent years. Traditional essay writing is not as popular as it once was and is often replaced with short answer questions (SAQs). The advantage of SAQs over essays is that they allow a wider range of topics to be examined in a single paper, and the marking is often more objective. They test knowledge recall as well as application of knowledge and understanding of principles.

The questions themselves can take a variety of formats, for example writing notes on a subject, filling in blanks in a paragraph, selecting the appropriate response from a list or one-line answers. Questions often have many inter-related parts. SAQs are usually not negatively marked so it is worth attempting all questions. In most examinations the questions usually have equal marks allocated to them unless otherwise stated. This often gives you a clue as to how much detail is expected in an answer for a particular question. This book does not include a marking scheme, but most questions ask for a particular number of responses.

The aim of the book is to help candidates assess their knowledge and identify the areas where they need to read more, as well as providing valuable examination practice. It is intended to be used as a revision aid for students taking the undergraduate or postgraduate examinations in dentistry, such as BDS, IQE and MFDS. Common and popular topics have been covered but it was not possible to cover the entire scope of dentistry comprehensively in the book! We hope that you will find this book to be helpful and easy to use.

Good luck for the forthcoming exams.

**Kathleen Fan and Judith Jones**

# 1

# Child Dental Health and Orthodontics

**1.1**  Fill in the missing details about tooth formation in the table below.

| Tooth | Mineralization commences | Eruption | Root formation completed |
|---|---|---|---|
|  | Birth | 6–7 years | 9–10 years |
| Upper As |  |  |  |
| Upper 3s |  |  |  |
| Lower 5s |  |  |  |
| Upper Ds |  |  |  |
| Lower 8s |  |  |  |

## Answer 1.1

| Tooth | Mineralization commences | Eruption | Root formation completed |
|---|---|---|---|
| Upper and lower 6s | Birth | 6–7 years | 9–10 years |
| Upper As | 3–4 months in utero | 7 months | 1.5–2 years |
| Upper 3s | 4–5 months | 11–12 years | 13–15 years |
| Lower 5s | 2.25–2.5 years | 11–12 years | 13–14 years |
| Upper Ds | 5 months in utero | 12–16 months | 2–2.5 years |
| Lower 8s | 8–10 years | 17–21 years | 18–25 years |

**1.2**  (a) Name two conditions that may result in delayed eruption of primary teeth.

(b) Name two local conditions and a systemic condition that may delay permanent tooth eruption (different from your answer to question 1.2 (a) above).

(c) Is hypodontia more common in the primary or permanent dentition?

(d) How common is hypodontia in the primary and permanent dentition?

(e) Which sex is it most common in?

## Answer 1.2

(a) Any two of the following conditions:
- Preterm birth
- Chromosomal abnormalities, eg Down's syndrome, Turner's syndrome
- Nutritional deficiency
- Hereditary gingival fibromatosis

(b) Local conditions – any two of the following:
- Supernumerary teeth
- Crowding
- Cystic change around the tooth follicle
- Ectopic position of the tooth germ

General conditions – any one of the following:
- Cleidocranial dysostosis
- Chromosomal abnormalities (Down's syndrome, Turner's syndrome)
- Nutritional deficiency
- Hereditary gingival fibromatosis
- Hypothyroidism
- Hypopituitarism

(c) Permanent dentition

(d) The prevalence of hypodontia in the primary dentition is less than 1% and in the permanent dentition it is about 3.5–6.5% (DiBiase, 1971, *Dental Practitioner*).

(e) Is it more common in females.

**1.3** (a) What do you understand by the term 'infraocclusion' and how is it graded?

    (b) An 11-year-old boy presents with an infraoccluded lower second deciduous molar. What percentage of primary molars are affected by this condition?

- 3–5%

- 5–8%

- 8–14%

- 15–20%

    (c) How would you manage this problem?

    (d) When would you refer for surgical removal?

    (e) If there is a permanent successor and the second deciduous molar is still infraoccluded and is below the gingival tissue, what could have happened to the second deciduous molar? What will you need to consider after removal of the second deciduous molar?

## Answer 1.3

(a) Infraoccluded teeth are teeth that fail to maintain their occlusal relationship with opposing or adjacent teeth. They were previously called submerged or ankylosed teeth. Infraocclusion most commonly affects the deciduous mandibular first molars. It is graded as follows:

- Grade 1 – the occlusal surface of the tooth is above the contact point of the adjacent tooth.

- Grade II – the occlusal surface of the tooth is at the contact point of the adjacent tooth.

- Grade III – the occlusal surface of the tooth is below the contact point of the adjacent tooth.

(b) 8–14%

(c) Take a radiograph to see if there is a permanent successor. If there is one, it is likely that the infraoccluded second deciduous molar will exfoliate at the same time as the contralateral tooth, when the permanent successor starts to erupt.

(d) When there is no permanent successor and the tooth will probably 'disappear' below the gingival margin.

(e) The second deciduous molar may have ankylosed. Space maintenance will need to be considered after the extraction to allow eruption of the permanent molar.

**1.4** (a) A fit and healthy 12-year-old girl attends with her mother following an accident in which she fell off the apparatus at her gym club. She has banged both her upper anterior teeth. Examination reveals no extraoral injuries, but both the upper central incisors are mobile and the crowns are palatally displaced. What special tests would you carry out and why?

(b) The upper central incisors are fractured in the mid-third of the roots. What treatment would you carry out and how long must that treatment be done for?

(c) If the coronal portion of the tooth became non-vital what treatment would you carry out?

(d) If there were no root fractures, would your management have changed?

(e) If a dentoalveolar fracture had been diagnosed, would your management have changed and if so how?

**Answer 1.4**

(a) The following tests are recommended:
- Vitality tests of all upper and lower incisors as they may have been injured in the accident.
- Periapical radiographs or an upper standard occlusal view to see if the roots are fractured.

(b) Splint the teeth using a flexible splint that allows physiological tooth movement. A wire splint that is bonded to the injured teeth and one healthy tooth on either side of the injured teeth using acid-etched composite is easy to construct and well tolerated.

The splint must be kept in place for 2–3 weeks. Previous treatment regimens used rigid splints for 2–3 months; this is now thought not to give the best results.

(c) The pulp should be extirpated up to the fracture line. The root canal is filled with non-setting calcium hydroxide to encourage barrier formation coronal to the fracture line. The calcium hydroxide should be changed every 3 months until the barrier forms, at which point the coronal root canal should be filled with gutta percha, and the tooth kept under review.

(d) The teeth are mobile and palatally displaced so they must have undergone some type of displacement injury. These would still require flexible splinting, usually for 2–3 weeks.

(e) Dentoalveolar fractures are bone fractures and therefore require rigid splinting for at least 3–4 weeks.

**1.5** (a) What do you understand by the term 'behaviour management?'

(b) Name three types of communicative management.

(c) If a child is unable to tolerate dental treatment, drugs may be administered to help the child cope with the procedure. One way of drug delivery is inhalational sedation. What drug is commonly used with this method?

(d) Give two contraindications to the use of this drug.

(e) Name another sedative drug that may be used and the possible routes of delivery.

## Answer 1.5

(a) Behaviour management is a way of encouraging a child to have a positive attitude towards oral health and healthcare so that treatment can be carried out. It is based on establishing communication while alleviating anxiety and fear, as well as building a trusting relationship between the dentist/therapist and delivering dental care.

(b) Any three of the following:
- Non-verbal communication
- Tell, show, do
- Voice control
- Distraction
- Positive reinforcement

(c) Nitrous oxide

(d) Any two of the following:
- Sickle cell disease
- Severe emotional disturbances
- Chronic obstructive airways disease
- Cooperative patient

Drug related dependency and first trimester pregnancy are also contraindications to the use of nitrous oxide.

(f) Midazolam – oral, intranasal sedation.

**1.6** (a) A fit and healthy 15-year-old girl complains of a wobbly upper tooth. Examination reveals that the tooth is a deciduous upper left canine and the permanent canine is not visible. Describe how you would determine whether there is an unerupted permanent canine.

(b) You have a panoramic radiograph and a periapical view. Describe how you could use these images to determine the exact position of an unerupted tooth?

(c) Name two other combinations of radiographs that could be used to localise the tooth.

(d) What single radiograph could be taken to determine whether the canine is buccally or palatally placed?

**Answer 1.6**

(a) Clinical examination – the angulation of lateral incisors may give a clue. A buccally placed canine tooth may push the apex of a lateral incisor palatally leaving the lateral incisor proclined. Palpation of the buccal sulcus and palate may reveal a bulge, which could be due to an underlying tooth. Radiographs are the definitive method of determining presence or absence of the permanent canine tooth.

(b) By using the parallax technique. When two views are taken with different angulations, any object that is further away from the tube will move in the same direction as the tube. This can be carried out in either the vertical or horizontal plane. With these two radiographs the tube has shifted from a near horizontal position in the panoramic radiograph to a much higher angulation in the periapical. If the canine tooth appears lower on the panoramic radiograph than it does on the periapical view then it has moved with the tube and is palatally situated and vice versa. If the tooth does not move at all then it is in the line of the arch.

(c) Any two of the following:
- Two periapicals taken at different horizontal angulations
- A periapical radiograph and an upper occlusal radiograph
- An upper occlusal radiograph and a panoramic radiograph

(d) Vertex occlusal radiograph

**1.7** What are the treatment options for impacted permanent canines when the deciduous predecessor has been lost. Give an advantage and disadvantage of each option.

## Answer 1.7

| Treatment option | Advantage | Disadvantage |
|---|---|---|
| No intervention and monitor impacted canine tooth | Easy | Still no tooth in gap – need prosthesis |
| Removal of impacted tooth | No possibility of cystic change | Surgical procedure; damage to adjacent teeth/structures; no tooth in gap – need prosthesis |
| Surgical exposure with orthodontically assisted eruption | Tooth ends up in proper position with an intact periodontal ligament | Surgery; patient needs to wear an orthodontic appliance (usually fixed appliance); prolonged treatment; tooth may not erupt |
| Transplantation of canine | Quick, tooth immediately put in place | Surgery; tooth may become ankylosed; loss of vitality; long-term prognosis not as good as teeth that erupt normally |

**1.8** (a) What types of appliance are the Andresen appliance, Frankel appliance and twin block appliance? How do they work?

(b) What age group of patients are they most effective in?

(c) Which type of malocclusion is most successfully treated with these appliances? What skeletal effects are thought to occur?

(d) Name two skeletal and two dental changes that are reported to occur with the use of these appliances?

## Answer 1.8

(a) They are all functional appliances. A functional appliance is an orthodontic appliance that uses, guides or eliminates the forces generated by the orofacial musculature, tooth eruption and facial growth to correct a malocclusion.

(b) Growing children, preferably before the pubertal growth spurt as they use the forces of growth to correct the malocclusion.

(c) Their main use is to treat Class II malocclusions, especially Class II div I. However, they can also be used to treat anterior open bites and Class III malocclusions.

There is still confusion about the exact effects of functional appliances on growth. The effects are a combination of both dentoalveolar and skeletal. With respect to the mandible, it is has been said that the mandible is stimulated to grow and the glenoid fossa remodels forwards as the appliances pull the condylar cartilage forwards, beyond the glenoid fossa. It is also claimed that forward maxillary growth is inhibited.

(d) Skeletal changes – any two of the following:
- Restraint or redirection of forward maxillary growth
- Optimisation of mandibular growth
- Forward movement of glenoid fossa
- Increase of lower facial height

Dental changes – any two of the following:
- Palatal tipping of upper incisors
- Labial tipping of lower incisors
- Inhibition of forward movement of maxillary molars
- Mesial and vertical eruption of mandibular molars

**1.9** (a) What determine(s) the response of a tooth when force is applied to it?

(b) What changes are seen in the periodontal ligament when orthodontic forces are applied to teeth?

(c) Give five complications of orthodontic treatment.

## Answer 1.9

(a) The magnitude and duration of the force.

(b) Depending on the side:
- Tension side – stretching of the periodontal ligament fibres and stimulation of the osteoblasts on the bone surface, leading to bone deposition.

- Compression side – compression of blood vessels, osteoclast accumulation which result in resorption of bone and formation of Howship lacunae into which fibrous tissue is deposited.

(c) Any five of the following:
- Root resorption

- Enamel decalcification

- Gingivitis

- Trauma/ulceration from attachment

- Allergy from attachments, etc. (nickel)

- Relapse

- Incomplete treatment

- Loss of tooth vitality

- Patient dissatisfaction

**1.10** (a) In the current economic situation health providers need to show that orthodontic services are appropriately allocated. Name a commonly used index that categorises the urgency and need for orthodontic treatment.

(b) How many components are there in the index and what grades does this index incorporate?

### Answer 1.10

(a) The Index of Orthodontic Treatment Need (IOTN). This was developed to help determine the likely impact of a malocclusion on an individual's dental health and psychological well-being.

(b) The IOTN has two components: the dental health and the aesthetic components. The dental health component has five grades and looks at traits that may affect the function and longevity of the dentition with grade 1 indicating no treatment need and grade 5 very great need.

The aesthetic component attempts to assess the aesthetic handicap of the malocclusion and the possible psychological effect and as such is difficult to grade. This part of the index consists of 10 photographs scored 1–10 where score 1 is the most aesthetically pleasing and 10 the least.

With regard to treatment need:

- Score 1–2: no treatment

- Score 3–4: slight need

- Score 5–7: moderate/borderline need

- Score 8–10: definite treatment need

The average score of the two components may be used, or as is more commonly done, the dental health component is assessed first; if this is graded 4–5 then it is not essential to assess the aesthetic component. If the dental health component is graded 3 then the aesthetic score is taken into account. An aesthetic score of 6 or above indicates a need for treatment.

**1.11** (a) A 12-year-old girl complains of a 'gap between her upper central incisors' that she is getting teased about at school. Name four causes of a midline diastema.

(b) How would you determine the cause of the diastema?

(c) Once the potential cause of the diastema has been identified how should the patient be managed?

### Answer 1.11

(a) Any four of the following:
- Physiological (central incisors erupt first and a diastema may be present until the upper canines erupt)
- Small teeth in large jaw (including peg laterals)
- Missing teeth
- Midline supernumerary, odontome
- Proclination of upper labial segment
- Prominent fraenum (actual role is unclear although it is often cited as a cause)

(b) History and examination. In particular, look for:
- A prominent fraenum. Pull the lip to put the fraenum under tension and look for blanching of the incisive papilla
- Proclination of upper incisors
- Size of the teeth in the upper labial segment

Radiographs will help confirm if any teeth are missing or the presence of supernumerary teeth. A notch of the interdental bone between the upper central incisors is another sign of a prominent fraenum.

(c) Consider the following management options:
- If the upper canines are unerupted and the diastema is < 3 mm then reassess after eruption of the canines.
- If the upper canines are unerupted and the diastema is > 3 mm orthodontic treatment may be needed when the canines erupt to approximate the incisors.
- If the upper canines are erupted then the incisors will require orthodontic approximation or restorative treatment to reduce the gap.
- If there is a prominent fraenum, the patient should be referred for an opinion/treatment of the fraenum. Surgical treatment would involve a fraenectomy.

- If a supernumerary or odontome is present then refer for surgical removal.

- If teeth are missing, consider closing the midline diastema and a restorative option for the space created further laterally.

- If the upper labial segment is proclined, a full orthodontic assessment is needed to determine if it is treatable by orthodontics alone or may require surgical intervention at a later date.

- If the upper central and lateral incisors are very narrow with spacing then it may be possible to refer for restorative treatment to restore the teeth with composite, porcelain veneers or crowns to increase the width and minimise the gaps.

**1.12** (a) How common is cleft lip and palate in western Europe?

- 1:200 births

- 1:700 births

- 1:1000 births

(b) At what age do most units carry out closure of the cleft lip?

- Neonatal period

- 3 months

- 6 months

- 9 months

(c) At what age do most units carry out repair of the cleft palate?

(d) Name two dental anomalies that often occur in cleft patients?

(e) At what stage may orthodontic treatment be needed?

(f) What may need to be carried out to aid eruption of the maxillary canine on the cleft side and when would this be done?

## Answer 1.12

(a) 1:700 births

(b) 3 months

(c) Between 9 and 18 months

(d) Any two of the following:
- Hypodontia
- Supernumerary teeth
- Delayed eruption of teeth
- Hypoplasia

(e) In the mixed and/or permanent dentition:
- Mixed dentition – proclination of upper incisors may be necessary if they erupt in lingual occlusion, otherwise orthodontic treatment is better deferred until just prior to alveolar bone grafting. Orthodontic expansion of the collapsed arch and alignment of upper incisors is required prior to alveolar bone grafting.

- Permanent dentition – fixed appliances are usually required for alignment and space closure. Orthognathic surgery and associated orthodontic treatment is carried out when growth is completed. Patients classically have a hypoplastic maxilla with a class III malocclusion, and orthognathic surgery is considered for improvement in aesthetics and function.

(f) Alveolar bone grafting (grafting or placement of cancellous and/or cortical bone from another site, eg hip or tibia, to the cleft alveolus) is carried out to make a one-piece maxilla. The grafting is usually done between the ages of 8 and 11 years when the canine root is two-thirds formed, to provide bone for: the canine to erupt into; support for the alar base of the nose; provide an intact arch to allow tooth orthodontic movement; and aid closure of any oronasal fistula.

**1.13** (a) How does fluoride affect teeth prior to eruption?

(b) How does fluoride affect teeth after eruption?

(c) What are the possible consequences of fluoride overdose?

(d) Fill in the blanks in the table below to indicate the recommended fluoride supplement regimen for children.

| Age | Fluoride dose per day |
|---|---|
| 6 months –3 years | |
| 3–6 years | |
| Over 6 years | |

(e) Teeth start forming before the age of 6 months so why are fluoride supplements not given to younger children?

**Answer 1.13**

(a) Effects of fluoride prior to eruption:
  - The teeth have more rounded cusps and shallower fissures.
  - The crystal structure of the enamel is more regular and less acid soluble.

(b) Effects of fluoride after eruption:
  - Decreases acid production by the plaque bacteria
  - Prevents demineralisation and encourages remineralisation of early caries
  - Remineralised enamel is more resistant to further acid attacks
  - Can inhibit bacterial growth and glycolysis

(c) Possible consequences of fluoride overdose:
  - Dental effects – enamel fluorosis, mottling, pitting
  - Toxic effects – gastrointestinal

(d)

| Age | Fluoride dose per day |
|---|---|
| 6 months –3 years | 0.25 mg |
| 3–6 years | 0.5 mg |
| Over 6 years | 1.0 mg |

(e) Infants < 6 months of age do not have adequate renal function to excrete fluoride. Hence fluoride is contraindicated until children are at least 6 months old.

**1.14** (a) What are the factors that would put a child at high risk for developing caries?

(b) How would you carry out a diet analysis for a child?

(c) List four pieces of dietary advice that you would give to a parent/patient.

## Answer 1.14

(a) Social factors:
- Family belonging to a lower socioeconomic group
- Irregular dental attendance
- Poor knowledge of dental disease
- Siblings with high caries rates

Dietary factors:
- Easily available sugary snacks
- Frequent sugar intake

Oral hygiene factors:
- Poor plaque control
- No fluoride

Medical history factors:
- Reduced salivary flow, or reduced buffering capacity
- Medically compromised
- Physical disability
- Cariogenic medicine taken long term
- High *Streptococcus mutans* and *Lactobacillus* counts

(b) You need to ask the parents (carer) to record on a sheet the time, the food and the amount of everything that is eaten over a 3–4-day period. Try to include one day from the weekend as dietary habits are often different then.

(c) Encourage:
- Safe snacks (but beware of high-salt foods), eg nuts, fruit, bread, cheese
- Safe drinks – water, milk, tea with no sugar
- Tooth brushing

Limit:

- The frequency of sugar-containing food and drinks

- Sweets to mealtimes or one day a week

Avoid:

- Chewy sweets in particular

- Sweetened drinks in a bottle

Discourage:

- There is some controversy surrounding long term breast feeding, but breast milk has a higher lactose content compared with cows' milk. On demand breast feeding may give rise to caries, hence try to discourage it

Note: Always try to be positive and do not make the parent feel guilty.


**1.15** (a) What is meant by the terms balancing and compensating extractions?

(b) What is the likely effect of premature loss of a deciduous canine?

(c) Is the effect greater or less with the premature loss of a deciduous first molar than with a canine?

(d) What would you recommend in a crowded mouth requiring the unilateral loss of an upper canine?

(e) What is the effect of premature loss of deciduous second molars?

(f) Do you compensate or balance the premature loss of deciduous second molars?

**Answer 1.15**

(a) A balancing extraction is the extraction of the same or adjacent tooth on the opposite side of the same arch. A compensating extraction is the extraction of same or adjacent tooth in the opposing arch on the same side.

(b) The primary effect of early loss of deciduous teeth in a crowded mouth is localised crowding. The extent will depend on several factors, including the patient's age, extent of existing crowding and the site of the early tooth loss. In crowding, adjacent teeth will move into the extraction space, hence a centreline shift will occur with the unilateral loss of a deciduous canine.

(c) A centreline shift will occur to a lesser degree with the unilateral loss of a deciduous first molar compared with a deciduous canine.

(d) The unilateral loss of a canine should be balanced as the correction of a centreline discrepancy is likely to need a fixed appliance and prevention is preferable to dealing with the problem.

(e) The premature loss of deciduous second molars is associated with forward migration of the first permanent molars. This is greater if the deciduous second molars are lost before eruption of the first permanent molars, so if possible, delay extraction of deciduous second molars until the first permanent molars are in occlusion.

(f) Neither.

**1.16** (a) An anterior open bite can occur with which types of malocclusion?

(b) Give a simple classification of the causes of an anterior open bite.

(c) An anterior open bite caused by one factor is relatively straightforward to treat. Which factor is this?

(d) What other occlusal features may you see in this situation?

(e) How will you treat an open bite due to the factor in Question 1.16 (c)?

## Answer 1.16

(a) It can occur in a Class I, Class II or Class III malocclusion.

(b) Skeletal causes:
  - Increase in lower anterior face height (increased lower face height or increased maxillary to mandibular plane angle)

  - Localized failure of alveolar growth

  Soft tissue causes:
  - Endogenous tongue thrust

  Habits:
  - Digit sucking

(c) Digit sucking

(d) Occlusal features that may be seen in this situation:
  - Retroclined lower incisors

  - Proclined upper incisors

  - Unilateral buccal segment crossbite with mandibular displacement

(e) It is best not to make a big fuss of digit sucking. Most children grow out of the habit and the malocclusion usually corrects itself after several years. However, if there are other aspects of the malocclusion that need treatment, this should not be delayed. Various appliances may help to break the habit.

**1.17** (a) Name five ways in which fluoride is administered to children?

(b) Give an advantage and disadvantage of each of the methods you have listed.

| Method | Advantage | Disadvantage |
|--------|-----------|--------------|
|        |           |              |
|        |           |              |
|        |           |              |
|        |           |              |
|        |           |              |

## Answer 1.17

(a) Any five of the methods listed in the table in answer 1.17 (b) can be given here.

(b)

| Method | Advantage | Disadvantage |
|---|---|---|
| General water supply | Very cheap, available to everyone, does not rely on patient compliance | Not readily available in the UK as there is opposition to fluoridation; varies with where the child lives |
| Milk, eg school milk schemes | Cheap; not carrying out extra regimen | Not available to all children |
| Salt | Cheap, not carrying out an extra regimen | Not in the UK |
| Toothpaste | Daily delivery; not an extra drug as patient already using toothpaste | Relies on patient brushing teeth |
| Gel | High fluoride content | Relies on dental professional; care required not to ingest gel |
| Varnishes | High fluoride content; may result in arrest of early lesions; can use them to introduce children to dental care | Relies on dental professional; care required not to ingest varnish |
| Rinses | Can use as part of oral hygiene regimen | Not good for young children |
| Tablets | Topical and systemic effects; have to take a tablet | Relies on patient/parent compliance |

**1.18** (a) What types of pulp treatment are there for deciduous molars?

Briefly describe each type and when you would use them.

(b) How would you restore a tooth that had undergone a pulpotomy?

**Answer 1.18**

(a) Types of pulp treatment for deciduous molars:

- Vital pulpotomy – this is done when there is a carious exposure in a symptomatic vital tooth. The coronal pulp is removed and the remaining pulp stumps are dressed with formocresol or 15.5% ferric sulphate. This is usually a one-visit treatment and the tooth is restored.

- Non-vital pulpotomy – this is usually a two-visit treatment that is carried out when the pulp is non-vital or when there is infection. The coronal pulp is removed and a pledget of cotton wool with Formocresol or Beechwood creosote is placed in the pulp chamber and sealed for 1–4 weeks. The tooth is restored with a temporary dressing. At the next appointment the cotton wool is removed and the tooth is restored if the symptoms have subsided.

- Devitalising pulpotomy – this is done when anaesthesia cannot be achieved for a vital pulpotomy. A pledget of cotton wool with paraformaldehyde paste is sealed into the tooth for 1–4 weeks or an antibiotic/steroid type paste may be used instead for 1–2 weeks. At the next visit the coronal pulp is removed and the tooth restored as for a vital pulpotomy.

- Pulpectomy – in this treatment the entire pulpal tissue is removed. It is done when there is non-vital tissue in the root canals. The canals are cleaned and dried and filled with calcium hydroxide paste.

(b) With a stainless steel crown usually.

**1.19** (a) Select the most appropriate word to fill the blanks in this paragraph about development of the maxilla and mandible.

The maxilla is derived from the .............. pharyngeal arch and undergoes .............. ossification. Maxillary growth ceases .............. in girls than in boys. The mandible is derived from the .............. pharyngeal arch and is a membranous bone. The mandible elongates with growth at the condylar cartilage, at the same time bone is laid down at the .............. vertical ramus and resorbed on the .............. margin. Mandibular growth ceases .............. than maxillary growth and is .............. in girls than in boys.

1 First, second, third

2 Intramembranous, endochondral

3 Earlier, later

4 Anterior, posterior

(b) What is the difference between endochondral and intramembranous ossification? Give an example of where each occurs in the head.

**Answer 1.19**

(a) The maxilla is derived from the *first* pharyngeal arch and undergoes *intramembranous* ossification. Maxillary growth ceases *earlier* in girls (15 years and 17 years in boys). The mandible is derived from the *first* pharyngeal arch and is a membranous bone. The mandible elongates with growth at the condylar cartilage, at the same time bone is laid down at the *posterior* vertical ramus and resorbed on the *anterior* margin. Mandibular growth ceases *later* than maxillary growth and is *earlier* in girls (average 17 years in girls and 19 years in boys).

(b) Endochondral ossification occurs at cartilaginous growth centres where chondroblasts lay down a matrix of cartilage within which ossification occurs. This occurs at the synchondroses of the cranial base. Intramembranous ossification is the process in which bone is both laid down within fibrous tissue, there is no cartilaginous precursor. This occurs in the bones of the vault of the skull and the face.

**1.20** (a) List two localised and three generalised causes of abnormalities in the structure of enamel.

(b) What do you understand by the term enamel hypoplasia and how does it differ from hypocalcification?

(c) Name three disturbances of dentine formation.

(d) What do you understand by the term Turner teeth?

**Answer 1.20**

(a) Localised causes – any two of the following:
- Infection
- Trauma
- Irradiation

Generalised causes – any two of the following:
- Amelogenesis imperfecta
- Infections: prenatal (rubella, syphilis); postnatal (measles)
- At birth: premature birth; prolonged labour
- Fluoride
- Nutritional deficiencies
- Down's syndrome
- Idiopathic

(b) Hypoplasia is a disturbance in the formation of the matrix of enamel which gives rise to pitted and grooved enamel. Hypocalcification is a disturbance in mineralisation (calcification) of the enamel and gives rise to opaque white enamel.

(c) Any two of the following:
- Dentinogenesis imperfecta
- Dentinal dysplasia type I and II
- Fibrous dysplasia of dentine
- Regional odontodysplasia
- Ehlers–Danlos syndrome
- Vitamin D resistant rickets
- Vitamin D dependent rickets
- Hypophosphatasia

(d) This is caused by infection from a deciduous tooth affecting the developing underlying permanent tooth. It results in abnormal enamel and dentine.

# 2
# Restorative Dentistry

**2.1** (a) Name five causes of intrinsic discoloration of vital teeth.

(b) The appearance of discoloured teeth can be improved by methods which require tooth preparation and those that do not. Please name two of each.

(c) How would you remove extrinsic staining from tooth surfaces?

## Answer 2.1

(a) Any five of the following:
- Trauma resulting in pulpal death
- Fluorosis
- Tetracycline staining
- Amelogenesis imperfecta
- Dentinogenesis imperfecta

(b) Methods requiring preparation:
- Veneer
- Crown

Methods not requiring preparation:
- Bleaching
- Microabrasion
- Composite veneers

(c) Removing extrinsic stains:
- Polishing the surfaces with pumice slurry and water or prophylaxis paste
- Ultrasonic cleaners
- Bleaching

**2.2** (a) What do you understand by the terms primary dentine, secondary dentine and tertiary dentine?

(b) What is the difference between internal and external resorption?

(c) Are teeth with internal resorption likely to be vital or non-vital?

(d) Are teeth with external resorption likely to be vital or non-vital?

(e) Replacement resorption may result in ankylosis. What are the signs of ankylosis?

## Answer 2.2

(a) Primary dentine is formed before eruption or within 2–3 years after eruption and consists of mainly of circumpulpal dentine. It also includes mantle dentine in the crown and the hyaline layer and granular layer in the root.

Secondary dentine is the regular dentine that is formed during the life of the tooth and laid down in the floor and ceiling of the pulp chamber. It is a physiological type of dentine after the full length of root has formed.

Tertiary dentine can be divided into reparative and reactionary dentine, both of which are laid down in response to noxious stimuli. Reactionary dentine is laid down in response to mild stimuli whereas reparative dentine is laid down directly beneath the path of injured dentinal tubules as a response to stronger stimuli and are irregular.

(b) Internal resorption starts within the pulp chamber of a tooth. External resorption starts on the surface of a tooth, most commonly on the root surface.

(c) Internal resorption can only occur in vital teeth (or partially vital teeth).

(d) External resorption may occur on vital or non-vital teeth.

(e) An ankylosed tooth:
- Has a different sound from a normal tooth when it is percussed, often described as a cracked china sound
- Lacks periodontal membrane space on a radiograph
- Has no physiological mobility
- May become infraoccluded as the jaw grows around it

**2.3** Complete the table with regard to the Basic Periodontal Examination (BPE) using the options given below.

| Code | Finding on probing | Treatment |
|---|---|---|
| 0 | | No need for periodontal treatment |
| 1 | | |
| 2 | | |
| 3 | Coloured area partly visible | |
| 4 | | |

Findings

- Coloured area of probe is completely visible, no calculus and no gingival bleeding

- Coloured area completely disappears indicating probing depth of > 3.5 mm but < 5.5 mm

- Coloured area is completely visible, no calculus but bleeding on probing

- Coloured area is completely visible; supra- or subgingival calculus detected or overhanging restorations

Treatment

- Oral hygiene instruction (OHI); elimination of plaque retentive areas; scaling and root surface debridement

- Complex treatment, referral to a specialist may be necessary

- OHI

- OHI; elimination of plaque retentive areas; scaling and root surface debridement

## Answer 2.3

| Code | Finding on probing | Treatment |
|------|-------------------|-----------|
| 0 | Coloured area of probe is completely visible, no calculus and no gingival bleeding | No need for periodontal treatment |
| 1 | Coloured area is completely visible, no calculus but bleeding on probing | OHI |
| 2 | Coloured area is completely visible; supra- or subgingival calculus detected or overhanging restorations | OHI; elimination of plaque retentive areas; scaling and root surface debridement |
| 3 | Coloured area partly visible | OHI; elimination of plaque retentive areas; scaling and root surface debridement |
| 4 | Coloured area completely disappears indicating probing depth of > 3.5 mm but < 5.5 mm | Complex treatment, referral to a specialist may be necessary |

**2.4**  (a) Name four general risk factors for periodontal disease.

(b) Name two localised risk factors for periodontal disease.

(c) Give two risk factors for gingival recession.

## Answer 2.4

(a) Any four of the following:
- Poor access to dental healthcare
- Smoking
- Systemic disease, eg diabetes
- Stress
- History of periodontal disease
- Genetic factors

(b) Any two of the following:
- Overhanging restorations and defective restoration margins
- Partial dentures
- Oral appliances
- Calculus

(c) Risk factors for gingival recession:
- Trauma – excessive toothbrushing, digging fingernails into gingiva, biting pencils
- Traumatic incisor relationship
- Thin tissues
- Prominent roots

**2.5** (a) How does fluoride affect teeth prior to eruption?

(b) How does fluoride affect teeth after eruption?

(c) What are the possible consequences of fluoride overdose?

(d) What is the recommended fluoride concentration in the water supply for optimal caries prevention?

(e) What do the following terms mean and at what dose do they occur?
- Safely tolerated dose
- Potentially lethal dose
- Certainly lethal dose

**Answer 2.5**

(a) Effect of fluoride on teeth prior to eruption:
- Teeth have more rounded cusps and shallower fissures.
- The crystal structure of the enamel is more regular and less acid soluble.

(b) Effect of fluoride on teeth after eruption:
- Decreases acid production by plaque bacteria.
- Prevents demineralisation and encourages remineralisation of early caries.
- Remineralised enamel is more resistant to further acid attacks.
- Thought to affect plaque and pellicle formation.

(c) Possible consequences of fluoride overdose:
- Dental effects – enamel fluorosis, mottling, pitting
- Toxic effects – gastrointestinal

(d) 1 ppm (in UK)

(e) Terms and doses:
- Safely tolerated dose – 1 mg/kg body weight. This is the level below which symptoms of toxicity are unlikely to occur.
- Potentially lethal dose – 5 mg/kg body weight. This is the lowest dose that has been associated with a fatality.
- Certainly lethal dose – 32–64 mg/kg body weight. At this dose survival of the individual is unlikely.

**2.6** (a) What is pulpitis?

(b) Fill in the blanks in the following sentences using the words in the table below. You may use more than one word/phrase if you think it is appropriate.

Reversible pulpitis is a ................. pain, set off by .................... . It is ................. localised and lasts for ................. .

Irreversible pulpitis is a ................. pain, set off by................. . It is ................. localised and lasts for ................. .

| Character | Sharp pain | Throbbing pain | | |
|---|---|---|---|---|
| Duration | Several minutes | Several seconds | Hours | Days |
| Localisation | Well | Poorly | | |
| Exacerbating factors | Sweet things | Hot/cold things | Biting | Spontaneously |

(c) What types of nerve fibres are there in the pulp?

(d) What special tests could you use to help diagnose reversible/irreversible pulpitis?

(e) What treatment is available for a tooth with irreversible pulpitis?

## Answer 2.6

(a) Inflammation of the pulp.

(b) Reversible pulpitis is a *sharp* pain, set off by *hot/cold things and sweet things.* It is *poorly* localised and lasts for *several seconds.* Irreversible pulpitis is a *throbbing* pain, set off by *biting or spontaneously.* It is *well* localised and lasts for *hours.*

(c) Nerve fibre types in the pulp:
   - A β fibres are large, fast conducting proprioceptive fibres.
   - A δ fibres are small sensory fibres.
   - C fibres are small unmyelinated sensory fibres.

(d) Special tests:
   - Percussion
   - Vitality tests
   - Radiographs

(e) Treatments for irreversible pulpitis:
   - Root canal treatment
   - Extraction

**2.7** (a)  Patients may have thermal sensitivity following the placement of a restoration. One theory for this is the thermal shock theory. However, another theory for the cause of thermal sensitivity is now more widely accepted – what is it called and what is it based on?

(b)  How can restorative techniques limit thermal sensitivity?

(c)  What are cavity sealers used for?

(d)  Give the types of cavity sealer.

(e)  What is meant by the term microleakage?

(f)  What are the consequences of microleakage?

**Answer 2.7**

(a) Theory of pulpal hydrodynamics

Fluid can move along dentinal tubules and when there is a gap between the restoration and the dentine, fluid will slowly flow outwards. A decrease in temperature leads to a sudden contraction in this fluid, and consequently increased flow, which the patient will feel as pain.

(b) When the thermal shock theory was widely accepted, insulating the cavity with a base material was used to prevent pain. Now that the hydrodynamic theory is more widely accepted the aim is to seal the dentine and increase the integrity of the interface between the dentine and the restorative material.

(c) To prevent leakage at the interface of the restorative material and the cavity walls, and to provide a protective coating to the cavity walls.

(d) Cavity sealers:

- Varnishes (eg a synthetic resin based material or a natural resin or gum)

- Adhesive sealers which also bond at the interface between the restorative material and cavity walls (eg glass ionomer luting cements)

(e) Microleakage is the passage of bacteria, fluids, molecules or ions along the interface of a dental restoration and the wall of the cavity preparation (Kidd 1976).

(f) Consequences of microleakage:

- Marginal discoloration of restorations

- Secondary caries

- Pulpal pathology

**2.8** (a) You are cutting a cavity in a vital upper first permanent molar. You have removed all the caries but then you create a small exposure of the pulp. How would you proceed?

(b) What is this treatment called?

(c) What are you hoping will happen to the tooth by carrying out this treatment?

(d) When would this treatment not be appropriate?

(e) What are the advantages of using rubber dam for dental treatment?

## Answer 2.8

(a) Management of an exposure during cavity preparation:

    **1**   If the tooth is not isolated already – isolate the tooth with rubber dam.

    **2**   Dry the cavity.

    **3**   Place calcium hydroxide over the exposure.

    **4**   Cover with cement/liner, eg glass ionomer.

    **5**   Restore as normal.

    **6**   Inform the patient.

    **7**   Arrange review.

Note: There has been some work using dentine-bonding agents to cover pulpal exposures although this is not universal practice at the present time.

(b) Direct pulp capping

(c) What may happen:

- A dentine bridge will form.

- The pulp will remain vital.

(d) Contraindications of pulp capping:

- Non-vital tooth

- History of spontaneous pain – irreversible pulpitis

- Evidence of periapical pathology

- Large exposure

- Contamination of the exposure with saliva, oral flora or bacteria from the caries

Also, the older the pulp the less the likelihood of success.

(e) Advantages of using rubber dam for dental treatment:

- Isolation and moisture control – especially important for moisture sensitive techniques, eg acid etching before composite restoration

- Prevention of inhalation of small instruments, eg during endodontic treatment

- Improved access to the tooth/teeth – no soft tissues, eg tongue in the way

- Patients do not swallow water and other irrigants

- Soft tissues protected from potentially noxious materials, eg etchant

**2.9**  (a) What restorative material is capable of adhesion to the tooth tissue without surface pretreatment?

(b) How may adhesion be improved?

(c) How does this material bond to tooth tissue?

(d) Besides the obvious advantage of being adherent, what other advantages are there of using this material?

(e) In what clinical situations is it used?

## Answer 2.9

(a) Glass ionomer

(b) Using a polyalkenoic acid conditioner.

(c) Glass ionomer bonds by:
- Micromechanical interlocking – hybridisation of the hydroxyapatite-coated collagen fibril network

- Chemical bonding – ionic bonds form between the carboxyl groups of the polyalkenoic acid and the calcium in the hydroxyapatite

(d) Other advantages of glass ionomer:
- It releases fluoride.

- Quick to use as limited pretreatment of the tooth surface is needed.

(e) Glass ionomer is used:
- As a permanent direct restorative material, suitable for deciduous and permanent teeth

- As a temporary restoration

- As a luting cement

- As a cavity lining or base

- As a core build-up material

- As a retrograde root filling material

- As a pit and fissure sealant

**2.10** (a) What do you understand by the term 'the smear layer?'

(b) Dentine can be treated with acid (or conditioned). What does this achieve?

(c) Why are primers needed during the process of creating an adhesive restoration?

(d) What do you understand by the term hybrid layer and where would you find it?

(e) What do dentine bonding agents do?

**Answer 2.10**

(a) When tooth tissue is cut, the debris is smeared over the tooth surface. This is called the smear layer and it contains any debris produced by reduction or instrumentation of dentine, enamel or cementum. It is calcific in nature or a contaminant that precludes interaction of restorative materials with the underlying pure tooth tissue.

(b) Within dentine, acid treatment removes most of the hydroxyapatite and exposes a microporous network of collagen. The smear layer is altered or dissolved. The bonding that results is diffusion based and relies on the exposed collagen fibril scaffold being infiltrated by the resin.

(c) The dentine surface after conditioning is difficult to wet with the bonding agents. The primer transforms this surface from a hydrophilic state into a hydrophobic state that allows the resin to wet and penetrate the exposed collagen fibrils.

(d) The hybrid layer is the area in which the resin of the adhesive system has interlocked with the collagen of the dentine, providing micromechanical retention.

(e) Dentine bonding agents:
- Form resin tags in the dentinal tubules.
- Stabilise the hybrid layer.
- Form a link between the resin primer and the restorative material.

**2.11** (a) What are the aims of obturating a root canal?

(b) Name the methods of filling a root canal with gutta percha?

(c) Name three causes of intra-radicular failure of a root canal treatment.

(d) Name two causes of extra-radicular failure of a root canal treatment.

(e) What are the indications for an apicectomy (surgical endodontics)?

## Answer 2.11

(a) Aims of obturating a root canal:
- To prevent reinfection of the cleaned canal.
- To prevent periradicular exudate from entering into the root canal.
- To seal any remaining bacteria in the root canal.

(b) Methods of filling a root canal with gutta percha:
- Single cone method
- Lateral condensation – warm or cold
- Thermomechanical compaction
- Vertical condensation
- Thermoplasticised gutta percha method
- Carrier based techniques

(c) Any three of the following:
- Necrotic material left in the canal
- Bacteria left in the root canal system (lateral or accessory canals)
- Contamination of the canal during treatment
- Loss/lack of coronal seal
- Persistent infection after treatment

(d) Two causes:
- Root fracture
- Radicular cysts

(e) Indications for an apicectomy:
- Infection due to a lesion that requires a biopsy, eg radicular cyst.
- Instrument stuck in canal with residual infection.
- Impossible to fill apical third of root canal due to anatomy or pulp calcification.

- Perforation of the root.

- Post crown with excellent margins but persistent apical pathology.

- Infected, fractured apical third of root.

**2.12** (a) What is acid etching of enamel?

(b) What acid is commonly used and at what strength? In what form are etchants produced (eg powder, liquid) and what effect do the different forms have on working properties?

(c) How long should the acid be applied for?

(d) What do you do after applying the etchant for the above length of time?

(e) What is likely to damage the etched enamel surface and reduce the efficacy of bonding?

(f) What do you understand by the term 'total etch technique' (or etch and rinse) and which acid would you use for it?

## Answer 2.12

(a) Application of a mild acid to the surface of enamel results in dissolution of about 10 μm of the surface organic component, leaving a microporous surface layer up to 50 μm deep. The surface is thus pitted, and the unfilled resin of the restorative material is able to flow into the irregularities to form resin tags that provide micromechanical retention.

(b) 30–40% Phosphoric acid is commonly used. Etchants come as gel or liquid, however, in the newer systems the etchant is combined with the dentine conditioner. The etch produced is the same with a gel or liquid but gels take twice as long to rinse away. Gels are less likely to drip onto areas where etching is not intended.

(c) Usually 15 seconds.

(d) Wash away the etchant with water for at least 15 seconds.

(e) Blood and saliva, and mechanical damage may occur by probing the area, rubbing cotton wool over it to dry it or by scraping across the surface with the suction tip or an instrument.

(f) The total etch technique involves using an acid to etch the enamel and condition the dentine at the same time. Commonly used acids include phosphoric acid (10–40%), nitric acid, maleic acid, oxalic acid and citric acid.

**2.13**  A 20-year-old fit and healthy woman attends your practice complaining of gaps between her upper anterior teeth. History and examination reveal that she has missing upper lateral incisors. List the treatment options in the table below. Give an advantage and disadvantage of each option. (Note: the number of rows in the table does not correspond to the exact number of treatment options, therefore all rows of the table do not have to be filled, or if you have more treatment options please write them below.)

| Treatment | Advantage | Disadvantage |
|-----------|-----------|--------------|
|           |           |              |
|           |           |              |
|           |           |              |
|           |           |              |
|           |           |              |

Answer 2.13

| Treatment | Advantage | Disadvantage |
|---|---|---|
| Orthodontic treatment to close the spaces | No artificial teeth needed; patient does not need restorative treatment to replace the teeth | May take a long time to complete; canines may not provide a good contact against the central incisors; bleaching and restoration of the canines may be needed to make them look more like incisors and recontouring of gingival margin |
| Removable partial denture | Quick; cheap; does not require removal of tooth tissue (although guide planes and rests may be needed) | Not ideal for young patients; removable; in the long term will need replacing. May compromise health of gingiva/teeth if oral health /diet not ideal |
| Adhesive bridges | Fixed tooth in place; no or minimal preparation of abutment teeth; good aesthetics | May debond; needs favourable occlusal clearance; in the long term may need replacing |
| Conventional bridge | Fixed tooth in place; good aesthetics | Requires destruction of adjacent teeth; in the long term may need replacing, impairs cleansability |
| Implants | Permanent solution; good aesthetics; like having a 'real' tooth | Costly; may need bone grafting; requires surgery |

NB. with the later 4 treatment options orthodontics may be required in conjunction.

**2.14** (a) Name three agents that are used for chemical plaque control and state how they are thought to work.

(b) Some antimicrobials (antibiotics) have been formulated in such a way that they are suitable for use within a periodontal pocket. Give four advantages of administering a drug in this manner and name one such antimicrobial?

## Answer 2.14

(a) Chemical plaque control:

- 0.12% Chlorhexidine digluconate – bacteriostatic at low doses and bacteriocidal at high concentrations. Bacterial cell walls are negatively charged due to the phosphate and carboxyl groups, but chlorhexidine is positively charged. Electrostatic charges cause the chlorhexidine to bind to the bacterial cell wall affecting the osmotic barrier and interfering with transport across the cell membrane. Unwanted effects are staining of teeth and altered taste.

- Quaternary ammonium compounds – cetylpyridinium chloride, benzalkonium chloride, benzethonium chloride. Net positive charge reacts with the negatively charged bacterial cell walls, causing disruption of the cell wall, increase in permeability and loss of the cell contents.

- Pyrimidine derivatives – Hexetidine (hexahydropyridine derivative). It has antibacterial and antifungal activity, affecting the rate of ATP synthesis in bacterial mitochondria.

- Phenols – antibacterial agents that penetrate the lipid components of bacterial cell walls. These also have an anti-inflammatory action as they inhibit neutrophil chemotaxis. Examples are thymol (Listerine), bisphenol (Triclosan).

- Sanguinarine – this is a benzophenathridine alkaloid and has antibacterial properties as it causes suppression of intracellular enzymes.

- Heavy metal salts – these are thought to work by binding to the lipoteichoic acid on bacterial cell walls and altering the surface charge which in turn affects the ability of the bacteria to adhere to teeth.

- Enzymes – lactoperoxidase, hypothiocyanate. These are thought to interfere with the redox mechanism of bacterial cells.

- Surfactants – these alter the surface energy (tension) of the tooth and this interferes with plaque growth.

(b) Any four of the following:

- Drug is actually delivered to where it is needed, not throughout the whole body
- High local drug concentrations can be achieved
- Fewer systemic side effects
- Overall lower doses of the drug need to be administered
- Drug delivery is not dependent on patient compliance
- Prolonged drug release

Example – any one of the following:

- Antimicrobials
- Tetracycline
- Metronidazole

**2.15** (a) What is a composite restorative material?

(b) List the types of composite restorative material you know in the table below. Give an advantage/disadvantage of each type.

| Material | Advantage | Disadvantage |
|----------|-----------|--------------|
|          |           |              |
|          |           |              |
|          |           |              |
|          |           |              |

(c) After placing a composite restoration how do you finish and polish it?

## Answer 2.15

(a) It is a type of restorative material made of a mixture of materials (hence the name): organic resin matrix, an inorganic filler and a coupling agent

(b)

| Material | Advantage | Disadvantage |
| --- | --- | --- |
| Traditional composites | Good mechanical properties | Surface roughness; difficult to polish |
| Microfilled resins | Very good surface polish | Poor wear resistance; unsuitable for load-bearing areas; high contraction shrinkage |
| Hybrid (blended) composites | Good mechanical properties; good surface polish | |
| Small particle hybrid composites | Good mechanical properties; very good surface polish | |

(c) Finishing involves shaping and smoothing the restoration to the anatomical form and polishing imparts a shine to the surface. The smoothest surface is achieved when composite is polymerised against an acetate strip with no polishing. This however, leaves a surface with a very high resin content that is not resistant to wear. For polishing:

- Diamond and carbide burs are used for gross finishing

- Rubber cups with abrasive materials of differing coarseness. The coarsest ones are used for gross finishing and the finer ones for polishing, They are good in areas with irregularities and the lingual surface of anterior teeth

- Flexible abrasive disks

- Finishing strips for interproximal areas

**2.16** (a) What are the risk factors for developing root caries?

(b) How would you manage a patient with multiple root caries?

(c) What restorative materials are commonly used for Class V lesions?

**Answer 2.16**

(a)  Risk factors of root caries:

- Exposure of the root surface (pocketing, gingival recession or attachment loss)

- Cariogenic diet

- Decreased salivary flow (medications, previous radiotherapy, drugs, diabetes, ageing)

- Poor oral hygiene – inaccessible areas (eg periodontal pockets); decreased manual dexterity; lack of access to dental healthcare or dental health is a low priority; removable prosthesis; restorations

(b)  Elimination of active infection (remove caries and place restorations), and preventive measures:

1  Identify any risk factors that can be corrected.

2  Oral hygiene advice.

3  Dietary analysis and advice.

4  Periodontal treatment as necessary.

5  Fluoride treatment in the surgery (eg Duraphat application) or home application (eg rinses).

6  Recall.

(c)  Glass ionomer, resin modified glass ionomer, composite and amalgam.

**2.17** (a) Nowadays it is possible to bond amalgam to tooth structure. Give four potential advantages of this over non-bonded restorations of amalgam?

(b) What other restorative materials can be bonded to tooth tissue?

(c) If you wanted to bond materials that are commonly used for anterior crowns how would they be pre-treated?

**Answer 2.17**

(a)  Any four of the following:

- Decrease in microleakage – less destructive of tooth tissue as traditional methods of creating retention for restorations involve removing tooth tissue to create dovetails, undercuts and grooves, etc.

- May limit the need for dentine pins.

- May increase fracture resistance of restored teeth.

- Transmits and distributes force better.

- There may be less postoperative sensitivity due to better sealing of the margins.

(b)  Materials that can be bonded to tooth tissue:
- Glass ionomers

- Composites

- Hybrid restorative materials, eg resin-modified glass ionomers, compomers

- Ceramics – using special cements

(c)  Pretreatment of anterior crowns:
- Conventional ceramics that are silica based are treated with hydrofluoric acid and ammonium bifluoride. They may also be sandblasted or air abraded. They are often treated with silane coupling agents.

- Alumina and zirconium oxide ceramics are surface roughened with air abrasion and then the surface is coated with a silicate.

**2.18** (a) What materials are commonly used for primary impressions for complete dentures?

(b) What broad groups can hydrocolloid impression materials and synthetic elastomeric impression materials be divided into?

(c) What do you understand by the following terms. Give one disadvantage of each.

- Mucostatic impression
- Mucocompressive impression

(d) What do you understand by the term selective mucocompressive impression?

## Answer 2.18

(a) Materials for primary impressions:
- Alginate
- Compound – thermoplastic
- Impression putty

(b) Hydrocolloids can be divided into: reversible (agar) and irreversible (alginate). Synthetic elastomeric impression materials can be divided into:
- Elastomers
- Polysulphides
- Polyethers
- Silicones (addition cured/condensation cured)

(c) A mucostatic impression is an impression taken with the mucosa in its resting state. It provides a good fit at rest and therefore good retention, ie most of the time but when the patient chews the denture will tend to rock around the most incompressible areas, eg a palatine torus. A mucocompressive impression is an impression taken when the denture-bearing area is subjected to compressive force. This results in a denture that is maximally stable during function but not at rest.

(d) This is an impression taken with only certain areas of the denture-bearing area being subjected to the compressive force.

**2.19** (a) What is meant by the terms RVD and OVD and what is their significance?

(b) Name one way of measuring the RVD or the OVD?

(c) In which patients is it important to measure the OVD?

(d) What factors may affect the jaw position at rest?

**Answer 2.19**

(a) RVD is resting vertical dimension. It is a measure of the vertical height of the patient's lower face and is measured as the distance between two arbitrary points – one related to the maxilla and the other to the mandible with the patient at rest. OVD is the occlusal vertical dimension. It is a similar measure to that mentioned above, but is taken with the patient's teeth in occlusion. The difference between the two measurements gives the freeway space, which is the vertical gap between the patient's teeth at rest.

(b) Any one of the following:
- Willis gauge to measure between two points on the face (eg nose and chin)

- Willis gauge to measure between the pupil of the eye and the mouth and then compare this with the distance between the base of the nose and the inferior border of the chin.

- Using two dots on two points on the face (eg nose and chin)

- Swallowing, which is thought to show the rest vertical dimension

- Phonetic methods

- Appearance

(c) Those patients with partial dentures and no natural teeth occluding, and patients with complete dentures or when changing the OVD of a worn dentition.

(d) What factors may affect the rest jaw position?
- Stress

- Head posture

- Pain

- Age

- Neuromuscular disorders

- Bruxism

**2.20** (a) What do you understand by the following terms:

- Group function
- Canine guidance
- Balanced occlusion

(b) Which would you try to create in a complete denture case?

(c) What is the difference between balanced occlusion and balanced articulation?

(d) When trying to achieve the correct occlusion in a complete denture case what factors will affect the occlusion in protrusive movements?

(e) What do you understand by the term lateral compensating curve and how does it affect the set up of complete denture teeth?

## Answer 2.20

(a) Group function means that during lateral excursions there is contact between several upper and lower teeth on the working side and no contacts on the non-working side. Canine guidance means that during lateral excursions there is contact between upper and lower canine teeth on the working side only and no contact on the non-working side. Balanced occlusion means simultaneous contacts between opposing artificial teeth on both sides of the dental arch.

(b) Balanced occlusion

(c) Balanced articulation is simultaneous contact of opposing teeth in central and eccentric positions as the mandible moves, ie it is a dynamic relationship whereas balanced occlusion is a static situation.

(d) Factors affecting the occlusion in protrusive movements:
- Incisor guidance angle
- Cusp angles of the posterior teeth
- Condylar guidance angles
- Orientation of the occlusal plane
- Prominence of the compensating curve

(e) During lateral excursions the mandible does not move in a horizontal plane only. There are vertical components to the movement due to the condylar guidance angle and the incisor guidance angle. To achieve occlusion in lateral excursions when the mandible and lower denture carry out these tipping movements the upper teeth need to be inclined buccally so that the occlusal planes of the teeth lie on a curve (viewed in the coronal plane). This is analogous to the Monson curve in the natural dentition.

**2.21** (a) Give three advantages and three disadvantages of an immediate denture.

(b) What do the terms flanged and open face mean with respect to an immediate upper complete denture? Give an advantage and disadvantage of each.

(c) If you wanted to adjust the fit of an immediate denture in the future what methods can you use?

**Answer 2.21**

(a) Advantages – any three of the following:
- Patient is never without teeth and so there are psychological advantages.
- Aesthetics – patient is never without teeth.
- Artificial teeth can be set in the same position as the natural ones.
- Soft tissue support.
- Easier to register jaw relations as they are taken when the patient had teeth.
- Bleeding easier to control after extractions

Disadvantages – any three of the following:
- Denture may not fit after extraction.
- Will need relining/copying or remaking.
- Will not fit when the alveolus remodels
- Unable to try-in.
- May need many visits for adjustment.

(b) Flanged means that the denture has a flanged periphery, like a normal complete denture. The advantage is that retention is good and will make future adjustments easier. The disadvantage is that the lip may be over supported/ appear too bulbous. Open faced means that there is no buccal flange and the denture teeth sit at the edge of the extraction sockets of the natural teeth. The advantage is that it can be used when there are large undercuts, it often has good aesthetics initially, but the retention is poor and when resorption occurs a gap appears between the gingival margin of the denture teeth and the mucosa.

(c) Methods to adjust the fit of an immediate denture:
- Relining
- Rebasing
- Copy dentures
- Total remake

**2.22** What is meant by the term altered cast technique? Explain the theory behind it. What stages are involved in carrying it out and in what situation could you use it?

## Answer 2.22

When a patient wears a denture with a free end saddle(s) (FES) supported by both tooth and soft tissue there is a risk that when a load is applied to the saddle (eg during function) the underlying mucosa will compress and the saddle will move. The part of the denture supported by the teeth will only move as much as the periodontal ligament of the teeth moves and so this differential movement will cause the denture to rotate. To overcome this an impression of the FES area is taken with the mucosa compressed so that minimal displacement will occur with loading and this reduces the rotation effect. However, overcompression of the soft tissues must be avoided as this can lead to either displacement of the denture when the tissues try to recover or to pressure necrosis of the mucosa.

This technique of taking a special mucocompressive impression of just the FES area(s) is known as the altered cast technique (of Applegate). The idea is to compensate for the difference in degree of support offered by the mucosa and the teeth.

Method:

1 The denture framework has base plates attached to the FES area. These are relieved to allow about 2 mm of space between them and the mucosa.

2 An impression is taken of the FES area with pressure applied only to the tooth supported part of the denture and no pressure applied over the FES.

3 The original working master cast is sectioned to remove the FES area.

4 The denture framework is reseated onto the cast and the FES impression area cast up.

**2.23** (a) What is a dental surveyor and what is the objective of surveying the diagnostic cast?

(b) What is a dental articulator?

(c) How would you classify articulators.

(d) What is a facebow and what is it used for?

**Answer 2.23**

(a) A dental surveyor is an instrument that is used to determine the relative parallelism of two or more surfaces of the teeth or other parts of the cast of a dental arch. The objectives of surveying the diagnostic cast are to identify:
- The most desirable path of insertion that will eliminate or minimise interference to placement and removal.
- Tooth and tissue undercuts.
- Tooth surfaces that are, or need to be parallel so that they act as guide planes during insertion and removal.
- And measure areas of teeth that may be used for retention.
- Whether tooth and bony areas of interference need to be eliminated surgically by selecting different paths of insertion.
- Undesirable tooth undercut that needs to be avoided, blocked out or eliminated.
- Potential sites for occlusal rests and where they need to be prepared.

(b) It is an instrument that is used to reproduce jaw relationships and movements of the lower jaw relative to the upper. Casts of both upper and lower jaws are mounted on the articulator.

(c) Classification of articulators:
- Hinge articulator
- Average value articulator
- Adjustable articulator – simple adjustable; fully adjustable

(d) A facebow is an instrument that measures the relationship of either the maxillary or mandibular arch to the intercondylar axis and is used to transfer these measurements to an articulator. This means that the articulated casts will have the same relationship to the hinge axis of the articulator as the teeth with the intercondylar axis.

**2.24** (a) Name five muscles whose movements may affect the peripheral flanges of a complete denture.

(b) Where is the posterior margin of an upper complete denture usually situated?

- Anterior to the fovea palatinae

- Posterior to the fovea palatinae

(c) What is a post-dam and what function does it perform?

(d) Where is it usually positioned?

(e) What do you understand by the term 'neutral zone?'

## Answer 2.24

(a) Any five of the following:
- Geniohyoid
- Orbicularis oris
- Mentalis
- Mylohyoid
- Buccinator
- Palatopharyngeus
- Palatoglossus

(b) Location of the posterior margin of the upper complete denture:
- Anterior to the fovea palatinae

(c) A post-dam is a raised lip on the posterior border of the fit surface of an upper complete denture. It compresses the palatal soft tissue to form a border seal.

(d) It usually lies at the junction of the non-moveable hard palate (anteriorly) and the moveable soft palate (posteriorly).

(e) The area between the tongue, lips and cheeks where the displacing forces of the muscles is minimal. It is the ideal area into which a prosthesis should be placed to minimise displacing forces.

**2.25** (a) What is the Kennedy classification for partially edentulous arches?

(b) What Kennedy classification does this charting fit into?

| | |
|---|---|
| 4321 | 123 |
| 54321 | 12347 |

(c) What are the stages in designing a partial denture?

(d) What is meant by the term direct retainer in a partial denture?

(e) Name the two broad classes of clasps.

(f) Clasps do not work in isolation, but are often termed as being part of a clasp unit. What else is incorporated into a clasp unit?

(g) Why are these other features needed?

**Answer 2.25**

(a) Kennedy classification:
- Class I – bilateral edentulous areas located posterior to the natural teeth
- Class II – unilateral edentulous areas located posterior to the remaining natural teeth
- Class III – a unilateral edentulous area with natural teeth remaining both anterior and posterior (bounded saddle)
- Class IV – a single, but bilateral (crossing the midline) edentulous area located anterior to the remaining natural teeth

Once the classification has been decided each additional edentulous gap is indicated by a modification number. Class IV does not have modifications.

(b) Example classification:
- Upper – Kennedy Class I
- Lower – Kennedy Class II modification 1

(c) Stages in designing a partial denture:
1 Outline the saddle areas.
2 Place occlusal rests seats.
3 Place clasps for direct retention.
4 Place the indirect retainers.
5 Connect the denture.

(d) Any element of a partial denture that provides resistance to movement of the denture away from the supporting tissues is a direct retainer.

(e) Clasps may be:
- Gingivally approaching
- Occlusally approaching

(f) A clasp unit also has:

- Some form of support, usually an occlusal rest.

- Some form of reciprocation.

(g) Support will allow loads to be transferred along the long axis of teeth. It will also enable the clasp arm to be accurately located in the undercut on the tooth. Reciprocation is needed as all clasps on teeth must be balanced by something on the opposite surface to act as a balance. This will prevent inadvertent force being applied to a tooth in one direction only and acting like an orthodontic appliance.

**2.26** (a) Copy dentures are sometimes indicated for patients. In what situations would these be made?

(b) What are the advantages of making a set of copy dentures?

(c) Briefly describe the stages in making a set of copy dentures.

**Answer 2.26**

(a) Indications for copy dentures:
- Occlusal wear on a set of previously successful complete dentures.
- Need for replacement of the denture base material.
- Patient was initially given immediate dentures and they need to be replaced.
- Patient has a set of complete dentures that they have been happy with but are now unretentive/worn, especially elderly patients who may find it hard to adapt to a completely new set of dentures.
- To make a spare set of dentures.
- If a patient has had problems with previous dentures it is advisable to copy the set that they like the most.

(b) Advantages:
- Simple clinical steps, quicker than starting from scratch.
- Reduced number of laboratory steps: no special trays needed; no record blocks needed.
- Patient is never without their denture.
- Original dentures are not altered in any way.
- More predictable patient acceptance.

(c) Steps for making copy dentures (one method – others are available):
1 Alginate impressions are taken of the dentures in boxes.
2 The dentures are given back to the patient.
3 In the lab the alginate moulds are poured up in self-curing acrylic bases.
4 The copy dentures are now assessed and adjusted as necessary by the clinician and tried in the patient's mouth and used to take an occlusal record.
5 These are sent to the laboratory and articulated, and then denture teeth are set up.

6 The copy dentures are used as special trays and impressions are taken of the fit surface.

7 In the laboratory the copy dentures are converted into heat-cured acrylic dentures.

**2.27** (a) Fill in the blanks from the following list of words:

............ is tooth surface loss from non-bacterial ............ attack. Smooth ............ surfaces are seen with restorations standing ............ . Tooth surface loss of the ............ surfaces of the ............ incisors is seen in cases of gastric reflux and vomiting. ............ is physical wear of a tooth by an external agent and may result in ............ cavities at the ............ ............ is physical wear of a tooth by another tooth, and it commonly affects ............ and ............ surfaces. Abfraction lesions are thought to be due to a combination of ............ and occlusally-induced tooth ............ .

1 Erosion/attrition/abrasion

2 Mechanical/chemical /thermal

3 Plaque free/plaque covered

4 Low/proud/level

5 Buccal/palatal/interproximal

6 Lower/upper

7 Class III/class IV/class V

8 Gingival margins/occlusal edges/palatal surfaces

9 Flexure/wear/caries

(b) What could be the cause of severe erosion in a 16-year-old girl?

(c) What specialist treatment should she receive?

**Answer 2.27**

(a) *Erosion* is tooth surface loss from non-bacterial *chemical* attack. Smooth *plaque-free* surfaces are seen with restorations standing *proud*. Tooth surface loss of the *palatal* surfaces of the upper incisors is seen in cases of gastric reflux and vomiting. *Abrasion* is physical wear of a tooth by an external agent and may result in *class V* cavities at the *gingival margins*. *Attrition* is physical wear of a tooth by another tooth, and it commonly affects *occlusal* and *interproximal* surfaces. Abfraction lesions are thought to be due to a combination of *abrasion* and occlusally-induced tooth *flexure*.

(b) Vomiting – bulimia nervosa; less likely – gastric reflux or pregnancy. Most likely excessive fizzy drinks /cola consumption

(c) If you suspect that she has bulimia nervosa then that is outside the scope of management for a dental practitioner. She needs to be referred to her general practitioner for further assessment and possible referral on to a psychiatrist.

**2.28** (a) You need to carry out root canal treatment on a mandibular first permanent molar and a maxillary first permanent molar.

On the given diagrams of the occlusal surfaces of these teeth mark where you will expect to find the root canals.

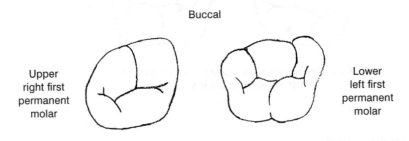

Buccal

Upper right first permanent molar

Lower left first permanent molar

Palatal/lingual

(b) How can you determine the working length of a root canal?

(c) What do you understand by the terms zip, elbow and transportation with respect to preparation of root canals?

**Answer 2.28**

(a)

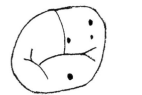 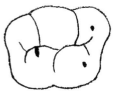

Black dots represent root canals – four in the upper
molar and three in the lower molar

(b) With the use of:

- An apex locator

- Working length radiograph with an instrument in the canal

(c) Zip and elbow are phenomena that occur due to instruments trying to straighten
out within a root canal. An hourglass shape is created with the narrowest part
being called the elbow and the zip being the flared apical part. The problem
with this type of canal shape is that it is difficult to fill the apical portion well.
Transportation is the selective removal of dentine from one area of the root
canal. This is done electively, for example when widening the coronal part of a
root canal, or can be an iatrogenic error.

**2.29** (a) What are the advantages of using a crown down method for preparation of a root canal?

(b) Why are root canals irrigated during preparation for root canal filling?

(c) Name two commonly used irrigants.

(d) Give five properties of an ideal root canal filling material.

## Answer 2.29

(a) Preparing the canal from the crown down gives better access. Flaring of the coronal part first removes restrictions and helps prevent instruments binding short of the working length. The coronal part is usually where most of the infected material is present. If this is removed and cleaned first it limits the possibility of spreading the infected material to the apical and periapical tissues. If you estimate the working length and then change the coronal part of the preparation it may inadvertently alter the length. Coronal preparation first allows irrigants to gain access to more of the root canal system.

(b) Physical removal of dentine by instruments does not get rid of all the bacteria in the root canal system. Irrigants reach the areas instruments cannot, and remove bacteria that would otherwise be inaccessible.

(c) Any two of the following:
- Sodium hypochlorite
- EDTA (ethylene diamine tetraacetic acid)
- Local anaesthetic solution
- Chlorhexidine
- Iodine-based irrigant
- Citric acid

(d) Any five of the following:
- It must be capable of sealing the canal apically, laterally and coronally.
- It should be radiopaque.
- It should be bacteriostatic.
- It should not irritate the periradicular tissues.
- It should be easy to handle, insert and if needed remove.
- It should be impervious to moisture.
- It should be dimensionally stable.

**2.30** (a) What is an overdenture and how does it differ from an onlay denture?

(b) Give four advantages of an overdenture.

(c) In what groups of patients would overdentures be useful?

(d) What factors need to be considered in choosing and preparing the abutment teeth.

## Answer 2.30

(a) An overdenture is a denture which derives its support from one or more abutment teeth by completely covering them beneath its fitting surface. An onlay denture is a partial denture that overlays the occlusal surface of all or some of the teeth. It is often used to increase the occlusal vertical dimension.

(b) Any four of the following:
- Preservation of the alveolar bone around the retained roots.
- Improved stability, retention and support.
- Preserved proprioception.
- Decreased crown-root ratio which reduces damaging lateral forces and reduces mobility in teeth with reduced periodontal support.
- Increased masticatory force.
- Psychological benefit of not losing all teeth.

(c) Overdentures are useful in:
- Severe tooth wear
- Patients with hypodontia
- Cleft lip and palate patients
- Motivated patients with good oral hygiene

(d) Factors to consider:
- The abutment should ideally be bilateral and symmetrical with a minimum of one tooth space between them.
- Order of preference: canine, molars, premolars, incisors.
- Healthy attached gingivae and periodontal support, minimal mobility.
- Dome root surface 2–4 mm above gingival margin.
- Root canal treatment may be required.

**2.31** (a) What is the definition of osseointegration?

(b) Give three situations when implants may be used in the head and neck?

(c) Give three patient-related factors that may affect the success of implant placement.

(d) What anatomical factors need to be considered with regard to implant placement?

(e) What would you see clinically if an implant failed?

(f) Success rate for single tooth implants are .............. than in edentulous patients. Success rate for implants in partially dentate patients are .............. than in edentulous patients. Chose the correct answer from the following: better, comparable, worse.

**Answer 2.31**

(a) A direct structural and functional union between ordered living bone and the surface of a load-carrying implant (Albrektsson *et al* 1981).

(b) Any three of the following:
- Single tooth replacement
- Bridge abutment
- Support for overdentures
- To support facial prosthesis and hearing aids
- Orthodontic anchorage

(c) Any three of the following:
- Oral hygiene
- Periodontal disease
- Previous radiotherapy
- Smoking
- Bisphosphonates

(d) Anatomical factors:
- Bone height
- Bone width
- Bone density or quality
- Proximity of inferior dental nerve
- Proximity of maxillary sinus
- Tooth position

(e) Clinical features of a failed implant:
- Mobility
- Pain

- Ongoing marginal bone loss

- Soft tissue infection

- Peri-implantitis

(f) Success rate for single tooth implants are *better* than in edentulous patients. Success rate for implants in partially dentate patients are *better* than in edentulous patients (Esposites *et al.* 721–764).

**2.32** (a) What are the constituents of dental amalgam?

(b) What are the gamma, gamma 1 and gamma 2 phases, and what is the importance of these different phases?

(c) What is the setting reaction of dental amalgam?

(d) What do you understand by the terms lathe cut particles and spherical particles? What is the significance of the different types?

(e) Why is it common practice to overfill a cavity and then carve it down?

(f) How should do you store waste amalgam?

**Answer 2.32**

(a) Constituents of dental amalgam:
   - Silver
   - Tin
   - Copper
   - Zinc
   - Mercury

(b) Gamma ($\gamma$) phase is $Ag_3Sn$; gamma 1 phase is $Ag_2Hg_3$; and gamma 2 phase is $Sn_7Hg$. The gamma 2 phase is the weakest part of the amalgam – it has the lowest tensile strength and is the softest of the phases. If the amount of gamma 2 phase can be limited in the final dental amalgam the resulting amalgam will be stronger.

(c) $Ag_3Sn + Hg = Ag_3Sn + Ag_2Hg_3 + Sn_7Hg$
   $(\gamma + mercury = \gamma + \gamma_1 + \gamma_2)$

   This is followed by $\gamma_2 + AgCu \rightarrow Cu_6Sn_5 + \gamma_1$: leaving little or no $\gamma_2$.

(d) Lathe cut alloy is made by chipping off pieces from a solid ingot of the alloy. This results in particles of different shapes and sizes. Spherical particles are made by melting the ingredients of the alloy together and spraying them into an inert atmosphere. The droplets then solidify into spherical pellets that are regular in shape and can be more closely packed together. This results in amalgam that requires less condensation force and results in increased strength of the amalgam.

(e) When amalgam is condensed the mercury rises to the surface of the restoration. To try to minimise the residual mercury left in the restoration it is usual to overfill the preparation and the excess mercury-rich amalgam can be carved away leaving the lower mercury containing amalgam which has a greater strength and better longevity.

(f) In a sealed container under liquid, usually x-ray fixative, solution.

**2.33** (a) What are dental ceramics made out of?

(b) What are the three technical stages in producing a porcelain jacket crown?

(c) Give one advantage and disadvantage of porcelain jacket crowns.

(d) How has the main disadvantage of porcelain jacket crowns been overcome?

(e) What does CAD-CAM mean in connection with ceramic restorations?

(f) Give three requirements of a metal-ceramic alloy.

## Answer 2.33

(a) Ceramics are made of feldspar, silica (quartz) and kaolin.

(b) The first stage is compaction. The powder is mixed with water and applied to the die so as to remove as much water as possible and compact the material such that there is a high density of particles, which minimises firing shrinkage. The next stage is firing. The crown is heated in a furnace to allow the molten glass to flow between the powder particles and fill the voids. The last stage is glazing, which is done to produce a smooth and impervious outer layer.

(c) Advantages – any one of the following:
- Excellent aesthetics

- Low thermal conductivity

- High resistance to wear

- Glazed surface resists plaque accumulation

Disadvantages – any one of the following:
- Poor strength and very brittle, so often fracture

- Firing shrinkage so must be overbuilt

(d) By fusing the porcelain to metal to produce metal ceramic restorations; by making reinforced ceramic core systems; and by creating resin-bonded ceramics.

(e) Computer assisted/aided design, computer assisted/aided manufacture.

(f) Any three of the following:
- High bond strength to the ceramic

- No adverse reaction with the ceramic

- Melting temperature must be greater than the firing temperature of the ceramic

- Accurate fit

- Biocompatible

- No corrosion

- Easy to use and cast

- High elastic modulus

- Low cost

**2.34** (a) What are the uses of dental cements?

(b) Give two examples of the types of material used for each purpose.

(c) Which zinc-based cement bonds to tooth substance?

(d) How should this material be mixed and why?

(e) Which cement should not be used under composite restorations and why?

(f) Which material is used for pulp capping and why?

(g) Which cement is thought to reduce sensitivity of a deep restoration?

## Answer 2.34

(a) Uses of dental cements:
- Luting agents
- Cavity linings and bases
- Temporary restorations

(b) Examples:
- Luting agents – modified zinc phosphate, zinc oxide and eugenol, zinc polycarboxylate, glass ionomer, resin modified glass ionomer, compomers, resin cements
- Cavity linings and bases – calcium hydroxide, zinc oxide and eugenol
- Temporary restorations – zinc oxide and eugenol, glass ionomer

(c) Zinc polycarboxylate.

(d) On a glass slab as it must not be mixed on anything that absorbs water, also a glass slab can be cooled and this will increase the working time.

(e) Zinc oxide and eugenol as the eugenol is thought to interfere with the proper setting of the composite material.

(f) Calcium hydroxide as it is extremely alkaline (pH 11), which helps with formation of reparative dentine. It is also antibacterial and has a long duration of action.

(g) Zinc oxide and eugenol is thought to reduce sensitivity due to the obtundent and analgesic properties of the eugenol.

**2.35** (a) What are the indications for anterior veneers?

(b) What materials are used for veneers?

(c) What would you need to check prior to advising placement of veneers?

(d) What is the long term prognosis of veneers and what would you warn the patient about?

(e) What is the thickness of the veneers?

(f) What are the key points during tooth preparation?

**Answer 2.35**

(a) Indications for anterior veneers:
- Discoloration of teeth
- For closure of spaces/midline diastema
- Hypoplastic teeth
- Fracture of teeth
- Modifying the shape of a tooth

(b) Materials used:
- Porcelain
- Composite (direct/indirect)

(c) Check the following:
- Is the discoloration enough to warrant treatment or is it so severe that it will not be masked.
- The patient's smile line –this helps determine which teeth need treatment if for aesthetic reasons only, placement of cervical margin
- Is there enough crown present to support a veneer
- Any occlusal restrictions, eg edge to edge occlusion, imbrication
- Any parafunctional activities
- Is there an alternative option, eg bleaching

(d) May require replacement in the long term (eg approximately 4 years for composite veneers) as a result of:
- Risk of chipping of incisal edge
- Debonding
- Need to keep good gingival health

(e) Usually 0.5–0.7 mm

(f) Key points during tooth preparation:

- Tooth reduction labially – depth cuts are helpful.

- Chamfer finish line is helpful for the technician.

- Margin – slightly supragingival unless discoloration, then margin can be subgingival.

- Extend into embrasure but short of contact point.

- Incisally either chamfer or wrap over onto palatal surface.

**2.36** (a) What is the function of a post and core?

(b) What is important to check prior to placement of a post and why?

(c) What is the ideal length of the post?

(d) Give a classification of a post and core system.

(e) What are the ideal characteristics of a post?

(f) What measures can be taken to avoid post perforation?

(g) How would you manage a post perforation?

## Answer 2.36

(a) Provides support and retention for the restoration and distributes stresses along the root.

(b) The condition of the orthograde root filling and the apical condition as placement of the post will make it difficult to redo the root canal filling so if necessary repeat orthograde root canal treatment.

(c) Ideal length is at least the length of the crown; approximately two-thirds of the canal length; and the apical seal must not be disturbed so at least 4 mm of well-condensed gutta percha should be left.

(d) Classification of post and core system:
   - Prefabricated or custom made
   - Parallel sided or tapered
   - Threaded, smooth or serrated

(e) A post should:
   - Have adequate length
   - Be as parallel as possible
   - Have a roughened or serrated surface
   - Not rotate in the root canal

(f) Careful choice of post:
   - Avoid large diameter post in small tapered roots, instead used tapered post and cement passively
   - Avoid long post in curved roots
   - Avoid threaded post which will increase internal stress within root canal

(g) Depends on the location of the perforation. If it is in the coronal third try to incorporate into the design of the post crown, eg diaphragm post and core preparation. For a minimal perforation in the middle third seal, the perforation (eg lateral condensation) and reposition the post. For a perforation in the apical two-thirds, use a surgical approach to try to reduce the exposed post and seal the perforation. If attempting repair of perforations, the use of MTA – mineral trioxide aggregate – would be preferable. Due to the poor long-term prognosis, extraction and implant placement may be favoured.

**2.37** (a) When are posterior crowns used?

(b) What are the principles of tooth preparation for a posterior crown?

(c) How much tooth reduction is required for different materials used for posterior crowns?

(d) What features affect the retention and resistance form of the crown preparation? Give three for each form.

(e) What are the advantages of partial coverage crown over full coverage crown?

**Answer 2.37**

(a) Post crowns are used for:
- Bridge abutments.
- Restoring endodontically treated teeth.
- Repairing tooth substance lost due to extensive caries/remaining tooth substance requires protection.
- Fractured teeth.
- Situations in which it is difficult to produce a reasonable occlusal form in a plastic material.

(b) Principles of tooth preparation:
- Remove enough tooth substance to allow adequate thickness of material (see below).
- Develop adequate retention and resistance form.
- Marginal integrity, supragingival and onto sound tooth where possible.

(c) Tooth reduction required:
- Full veneer gold crown – 1.5 mm on functional cusp, 1 mm elsewhere.
- Porcelain fused to metal crown – same tooth reduction as for gold crown except where porcelain coverage is required where more tooth substance must be removed.
- Occlusal reduction – metal occlusal surface requires same tooth reduction as for gold crown.
- All porcelain – occlusal surface 2 mm supporting cusps and 1.5 mm non- supporting cusps; buccal reduction 1.2–1.5 mm; margins 1.2–1.5 mm; shoulder: if porcelain to tooth margin otherwise chamfer finish as for gold crown.

(d) Retention relies on the height, diameter and taper of the preparation. It will also be increased by the placement of boxes, groves, pins and surface texture. Resistance relies on taper of preparation, height to diameter ratio, correctly aligned and positioned grooves and boxes.

(e) Advantages of partial coverage crown:

- Preservation of tooth structure

- Less pulpal damage

- Margins more likely to be supragingival

- Remaining tooth substance can act as a guide for the technician

**2.38** (a) A 21-year-old woman presents with gingival recession affecting the lower incisors. How will you manage this?

(b) If the recession is mild on all except the lower left lateral incisor how would you proceed?

(c) What are the possible causes of gingival recession?

(d) If the gingival recession continues on the lower left lateral incisor what other options may you consider?

(e) Where is the free graft often taken from?

## Answer 2.38

(a) Take a thorough history:
- Present concerns, sensitivity
- History of presenting complaint
- Dental history
- Toothbrushing history, frequency and duration
- Any previous orthodontic treatment

Then examination should include assessment of presence of plaque, recession, probing depth, bleeding, amount of attached gingivae, presence of functional gingivae, tooth mobility, vitality testing, occlusion, oral hygiene technique and instructions.

(b) Target traumatic tooth brushing and improve plaque control; monitor the progression with clinical measurements, photographs; and treat sensitivity. Take impression for study models.

(c) Causes of gingival recession:
- Traumatic toothbrushing
- Incorrect toothbrushing technique
- Abrasive toothpaste
- Traumatic occlusion/incisor relationship
- Tooth out of arch
- Orthodontic movement of tooth labially
- Habits such as rubbing of gingivae with fingernail, pen, etc.

(d) Mucogingival surgery to correct recession by a:
- Lateral pedicle graft
- Double papilla flap

- Coronally repositioned flap (these can be sewn with a interpositional graft)
- Free gingival graft to provide a wider and functional zone of attached gingivae
- Thin acrylic gingival veneer/stent (rarely used)

(e) Palate

**2.39** (a) Give six clinical features of necrotising ulcerative gingivitis.

(b) What organisms are implicated?

(c) What are the risk factors for necrotising ulcerative gingivitis?

(d) How would you treat it?

## Answer 2.39

(a) Any six of the following:
- Painful yellowish white ulcer
- Initially involve the interdental papillae
- Spread to involve the labial and lingual marginal gingivae
- Metallic taste
- Regional lymphadenopathy
- Fever
- Malaise
- Poor oral hygiene
- Sensation of teeth being wedged apart
- Fetor oris

(b) Mixed picture: fuso-spirochaetal organisms (*Borrelia vincentii*, *Fusobacterium fusiformis*) and Gram-negative anaerobes including *Porphyromonas*, *Treponema* species, *Selenomonas* species and *Prevotella* species.

(c) Risk factors are:
- Poor oral hygiene
- Pre-existing gingivitis
- Smoking
- Stress
- Malnourishment and debilitation
- Human immunodeficiency virus (HIV) infection

(d) Treatment of necrotising ulcerative gingivitis:
- Local measures
- Oral hygiene instruction

- Debridement

- Chemical plaque control, eg chlorhexidine

- Metronidazole 200–400 mg three times daily for 3 days if systemically unwell

- Advice on management of risk factors, oral hygiene instruction, nutritional advice

**2.40** (a) How can you classify periodontal disease?

(b) Define localised juvenile periodontitis?

(c) How do you manage it?

(d) Give four indications for periodontal surgery?

## Answer 2.40

(a) Gingival disease:
- Gingivitis
- Necrotising ulcerative gingivitis (NUG)

Periodontal disease:

- (Aggressive periodontitis) Early-onset periodontitis (prepubertal, juvenile periodontitis)
- (Aggressive periodontitis) Rapidly progressive periodontitis
- Adult periodontitis
- Necrotising ulcerative gingivitis periodontitis
- HIV periodontitis

Alternative classification of Periodontal disease (Armitage GC, 1999)
- I – Chronic periodontitis
- II – Aggressive periodontitis
- III – Periodontitis as a manifestation of systemic disease
- IV – Necrotising periodontal disease
- V – Abscesses of the periodontium
- VI – Periodontitis associated with endodontic lesions
- VII – Development of acquired deformities and conditions

(b) An aggressive periodontitis occurring in an otherwise healthy adolescence, characterised by rapid loss of connective tissue attachment and alveolar bone loss. Usually localised to the incisors and first molars although it can be generalised.

(c) Management of juvenile periodontitis:
1 Oral hygiene instruction.
2 (Microbiology culture and sensitivity) MCS of subgingival flora.
3 Scale and root planing and/or access flap surgery.

**4** Antibiotics (usually responds to tetracycline).

**5** Consider surgical excision of pocket lining.

(d) There are no strict indications of periodontal surgery but in certain clinical situations it is more likely to be indicated:

- Pockets greater than 6 mm

- Pockets associated with thick fibrous gingivae

- Furcation involvement

- Mucogingival deformities or extensive periodontitis lesion requiring reconstruction or regenerative treatment

- Short clinical crown requiring increase in clinical crown height

- Gingival hyperplasia

# 3
# Oral Surgery

**3.1** (a) What does the term pericoronitis mean? Which teeth are most commonly affected by it?

(b) What are the signs and symptoms of pericoronitis?

(c) How do you treat acute pericoronitis?

## Answer 3.1

(a) Pericoronitis means infection of the tissue surrounding the crown of a tooth. The lower third molars are most commonly affected.

(b) Depends on the severity of the infection:

- Mild – swelling of soft tissue around the crown of the tooth, bad taste, pain

- Moderate – lymphadenopathy, trismus, extraoral swelling

- Severe – fever, malaise, spreading infection and abscess formation

(c) Treatment depends on the severity of the infection. Management of mild infection includes:

- Oral hygiene instructions such as cleaning around the tooth and operculum with chlorhexidine or hot salty water

- Relief of trauma from opposing tooth – grind cusps or extraction of the tooth

- Analgesics

- Antibiotics (Metronidazole)

Severe infection may need hospitalisation, intravenous antibiotics, removal of the lower third molar and/or incision and drainage.

**3.2** (a) What does the acronym NICE stand for?

(b) NICE guidelines gives specific indications for removal of wisdom teeth. List five such indications.

(c) What features on a radiograph would suggest that a wisdom tooth is associated with the inferior dental nerve?

(d) What specific information must be given to a patient prior to removal of an impacted lower wisdom tooth, which you would not give if you were removing an upper wisdom tooth?

## Answer 3.2

(a) National Institute of Health and Clinical Excellence

(b) Surgical removal of impacted third molars should be limited to patients with evidence of pathology such as (any five of the following):
- Caries
- Non-treatable pulpal and/or periapical pathology
- Cellulitis
- Abscess and osteomyelitis
- Internal and external resorption of the tooth or adjacent tooth
- Fracture of tooth
- Tooth/teeth impeding surgery or reconstructive jaw surgery
- Tooth is within the field of tumour resection

(c) Loss, deviation or narrowing of the 'tramlines' of the inferior dental canal, and a radiolucent band across the root of the tooth.

(d) Information specific to lower wisdom teeth: numbness/tingling of the lower lip, chin and tongue which may be temporary or permanent. This information needs to be given to the patient because of the possibility of damage to the inferior dental nerve or the lingual nerve during the procedure.

**3.3** (a) What do you understand by the term meal-time syndrome?

(b) Which gland does it affect most commonly and why?

(c) What investigations would you carry out if it affected this gland?

(d) How would you manage an acute episode?

## Answer 3.3

(a) Patients who have an obstruction in a duct of a major salivary gland often complain of pain and swelling in the region of that gland on smelling or eating food and also on anticipation of food.

(b) It most commonly affects the submandibular salivary gland because the saliva produced by this gland is a thick mucus-type, and the duct is long and has an upward course with a bend at the hilum.

(c) Investigations:
- Bimanual palpation
- Plain radiography – usually a lower occlusal view although a calculus may be seen on a panoramic radiograph.
- Sialography
- Ultrasound
- Scintiscanning

(d) Management of an acute episode:
- Encourage salivation, eg by massaging the gland
- Hot salty mouth baths
- Consider commencing antibiotics
- Arrange review for definitive treatment when acute symptoms have subsided

**3.4**    (a) A patient complains of an ulcer on their tongue. Which of the following features of the ulcer would make you suspect that it was malignant:

- Indurated

- Rolled edges

- Healing

- Pain

- Size

- A whole crop of ulcers present

- Present on the tip of the dorsum of the tongue

- Present on the lateral border of the tongue

- Healing

(b) Which groups of people are most likely to have oral malignancies?

- Children/young adults/older adults

- Males/females

(c) What are the risk factors for oral malignancy?

(d) What is the most common malignancy of the oral cavity?

(e) What treatment is available for the most common malignancy of the oral cavity?

## Answer 3.4

(a) Features suspicious of malignancy:
- Indurated
- Rolled edges
- Present on the lateral border of the tongue

(b) People most likely to have oral malignancies:
- Older adults
- Males

(c) Risk factors for oral malignancy:
- Smoking
- Alcohol consumption
- Intraoral use of tobacco products such as snuff
- Betel nut/pan chewing

(d) Squamous cell carcinoma

(e) Surgery:
- Excision and primary closure
- Excision and reconstruction

Radiotherapy:
- Surgery and radiotherapy (and/or chemotherapy) combined
- Other modalities
- Photodynamic therapy

**3.5** (a) What does the term 'internal derangement of the temporomandibular joint (TMJ)' mean?

(b) What might a patient with an internal derangement of their TMJ complain of? Please give the underlying reason for the complaint.

(c) If the internal derangement was unilateral, to which side would the mandible deviate on opening and why?

(d) If imaging of the TMJ were required, which type would be ideal?

## Answer 3.5

(a) A localised mechanical fault in the joint, which interferes with its smooth action.

(b) Patients may complain of:
- Clicking of the joint (displacement of the disc prevents the condyle from moving smoothly and if the disc and condyle 'jump' over each other, this is felt by the patient as a click or pop).

- Locking of the joint (the disc may be displaced and prevent the condyle from moving normally within the fossa. This may have the effect of locking of the jaw).

- Pain in the joint (may be due to the joint itself, and alteration in the synovial fluid has been suggested as a cause for arthropathy. There may also be associated muscle spasm which can cause pain).

(c) The mandible would deviate towards the side of the internal derangement. This is because the mandible is able to carry out the hinge movement normally, hence the mouth opens (usually about 1 cm). Further movement is usually due to translation of the condyle. If there is an obstruction on one side that condyle will not translate and move forwards. The other condyle continues to move in a normal manner and the midline moves towards the static condyle, ie the side with the internal derangement.

(d) Magnetic resonance imaging (MRI)

**3.6** (a) Which branch of the Trigeminal nerve is most frequently affected in trigeminal neuralgia?

(b) In which sex and at what age does this occur more commonly?

(c) If you had a patient with symptoms of trigeminal neuralgia who did not fit into the common demographic group, what other condition might they have?

(d) Give five features of the pain of trigeminal neuralgia.

(e) Name two types of medication that are effective in trigeminal neuralgia?

(f) Trigeminal neuralgia affecting the ID nerve of the mandibular branch of the Trigeminal nerve may be treated surgically. What procedures do you know that can be used on the distal (peripheral) aspect of the nerve?

(g) Less commonly neuralgia may affect another cranial nerve and patients may present with pain to their dentist. Which nerve is involved?

## Answer 3.6

(a) Mandibular > maxillary > ophthalmic

(b) Female > male, mid to old age

(c) Differential diagnosis:
- Multiple sclerosis
- A central lesion

(d) Any five of the following:
- Paroxysmal
- Trigger area
- Does not disturb sleep
- Excruciating pain
- Shooting
- Sharp, electric shock, burning character
- Short acting

(e) Any two of the following:
- Carbamazepine
- Phenytoin
- Gabapentin
- Lamotrigine
- Oxcarbazepine
- Baclofen

(f)
- Cryotherapy
- Alcohol injection
- Nerve sectioning

All the above procedures are done at the point where the nerve enters the mandible at the lingula.

(g) Glossopharyngeal nerve

**3.7** (a) What do you understand by the term 'dry socket?'

(b) Give five factors that would predispose a patient to getting a dry socket?

(c) How soon after the extraction does the pain usually start?

(d) How would you manage a patient with a dry socket?

## Answer 3.7

(a) It is the localised osteitis that occurs in a socket following removal of a tooth.

(b) Any five of the following:
- Smoking
- Oral contraceptives
- Difficult extractions
- Mandibular extractions
- Posterior extractions
- Single extractions
- Immunosuppression
- Bony pathology

(c) 2–3 days after the extraction.

(d) Steps in the management of dry socket:
1 Reassurance and explanation.
2 Give analgesics.
3 Debride the socket with chlorhexidine or warm salty water.
4 Gentle pack the socket with a dressing, eg Alvogyl.
5 Review if necessary.

**3.8** (a) What are the common signs and symptoms of each of the following conditions? Choose the most appropriate from the list below. Options may be used either once, or not at all.

1 Undisplaced unilateral fractured mandibular condyle

2 Orbital blow-out fracture

3 Bilateral displaced fractured condyles

4 Le Fort III fracture

5 Fractured zygomatic arch

6 Fractured zygoma

7 Fracture of the angle of the mandible

8 Dislocated mandible

    a Anterior open bite

    b Anaesthesia/paraesthesia of the infraorbital nerve

    c Anaesthesia/paraesthesia of the inferior orbital nerve

    d Limited eye movements especially when trying to look upwards

    e Trismus

    f Pain on mandibular movements but no occlusal alteration

    g Anaesthesia/paraesthesia of the inferior dental nerve

    h Anaesthesia/paraesthesia of the facial nerve

    i Cerebrospinal fluid (CSF) leak from the nose

    j Limited mandibular movement possible, but inability to occlude or open wide. The patient appears to have a class III malocclusion, with hollowing of the TMJ area.

(b) What do you understand by the term orbital blow-out? Which part of the orbit is most likely to fracture and why?

**Answer 3.8**

(a)    1    Undisplaced unilateral fractured mandibular condyle – pain on mandibular movements but no occlusal alteration

       2    Orbital blow out fracture – limited eye movements especially when trying to look upwards

       3    Bilateral displaced fractured condyles – anterior open bite

       4    Le Fort III fracture – CSF leak from the nose

       5    Fractured zygomatic arch – trismus

       6    Fractured zygoma – anaesthesia/paraesthesia of the infraorbital nerve

       7    Fracture of the angle of the mandible – anaesthesia/paraesthesia of the inferior dental nerve

       8    Dislocated mandible – limited mandibular movement possible, but inability to occlude or open wide. The patient appears to have a class III malocclusion, with hollowing of the TMJ area.

(b) Orbital blow-out means that the rim of the orbit is intact but some part of the bony orbital wall has been fractured. Usually the floor or the medial wall fractures as the bone is thinnest in these regions.

**3.9** (a) For each of the following conditions select the most appropriate medicine from the list below. Each option may be used either once or not at all.

1 Bell's palsy

2 Atypical facial pain

3 Acute pericoronitis

4 Post surgical pain relief

5 Angular cheilitis

6 Antibiotic cover for an extraction for a patient with a prosthetic heart valve

7 Prevention of post-surgical bleeding

8 Trigeminal neuralgia

- Ibuprofen 40 mg three times daily for 5 days
- Ibuprofen 400 mg three times daily for 5 days
- Carbamazepine 100–200 mg twice daily
- Prednisolone 0.5 mg/kg/12 hours for 5 days
- Aciclovir
- Miconazole gel
- Nortriptyline 10 mg continuing prescription
- Metronidazole 200 mg three times daily for 5 days
- Metronidazole 200 mg four times daily for 5 days
- Tranexamic acid mouthwash three times daily for 5 days
- Amoxicillin 3 g

(b) Name four local measures that can be used to control post-surgical bleeding?

## Answer 3.9

(a)  1  Bell's palsy – prednisolone 0.5mg/kg/12 hours for 5 days

2  Atypical facial pain – nortriptyline 10 mg continuing prescription

3  Acute pericoronitis – metronidazole 200 mg three times daily for 5 days

4  Post-surgical pain relief – ibuprofen 400 mg three times daily for 5 days

5  Angular cheilitis – miconazole gel

6  Antibiotic cover for an extraction for a patient with a prosthetic heart valve– amoxicillin 3 g

7  Prevention of post-surgical bleeding – tranexamic acid mouthwash three times daily for 5 days

8  Trigeminal neuralgia – carbamazepine 100–200 mg twice daily

(b)  Any four of the following:

- Apply pressure

- Administer local anaesthetic with vasoconstrictor

- Pack with haemostatic dressing, eg Surgicel

- Suture

- Bone wax

- Biting on a swab soaked with tranexamic acid, tranexamic acid mouthwashes

- Acrylic suck-down splint

**3.10** (a) What are the aims of management of a fractured mandible?

(b) What are the stages of managing a fractured mandible that needs active treatment?

(c) The most common mode of treatment of fractures of the mandible nowadays involves the use of mini-bone plates across the fracture site. Why is intermaxillary fixation often done along with this?

(d) Give three complications of a fracture of the mandible.

(e) What term is used to describe a fracture that involves both condyles and the symphyseal region, and what is the characteristic mechanism of injury?

## Answer 3.10

(a) Restoration of function and aesthetics

(b) Stages of treatment/management
  - Reduction
  - Fixation
  - Immobilisation
  - Rehabilitation

(c) Intermaxillary fixation is done to re-create the patient's original occlusion whilst the fractured bone ends are fixed together.The IMF also allows extra traction to be applied after the operation if needed.

(d) Any three of the following:
  - Non-union
  - Malunion
  - Infection
  - Malocclusion
  - Nerve damage

(e) Guardsman fracture – it is thought to occur when a patient falls on their chin (traditionally Guardsman fainting on parade – hence the name) or suffers a blow to their chin.

**3.11** (a) What signs and symptoms would make you suspect that you have created an oroantral communication following the extraction of an upper first permanent molar?

(b) If you have created an oroantral communication how would you treat it?

(c) If a root is pushed into the antrum how can a surgeon gain access to remove the root once the socket had healed?

**Answer 3.11**

(a) Signs and symptoms of an oroantral communication:
- A visible defect or antral mucosa visible on careful examination of socket
- Hollow sound when suction used in socket
- Bone with smooth concave upper surface (with or without antral mucosa on it) between the roots

(b) Management of an oroantral communication:
- Surgical closure of the defect by: approximating the palatal and buccal mucosa, but there is usually inadequate soft tissue; buccal advancement flap alone or with buccal fat pad; or palatal rotation flap.
- Advise the patient not to blow the nose for 10 days.
- Some surgeons prescribe broad-spectrum antibiotics, inhalation and nasal decongestants.

(c) By raising a flap in the buccal sulcus in the region of the upper canine/premolars and removing bone – known as a Caldwell–Luc procedure.

**3.12** (a) Fill in the blanks from the list of options below.

Bell's palsy is paralysis of the ............... nerve which results in a facial palsy.
It may be caused by a ................. infection particularly ................. .
Treatment involves a ................. course of ................., as well as
................. .

 1 Trigeminal/glossopharyngeal/facial

 2 Bacterial/protozoal/viral

 3 Herpes simplex/Epstein–Barr/bovine spongiform encephalopathy

 4 Short/intermediate/long

 5 Amoxicillin/prednisolone/gabapentin

 6 Augmentin/gentamicin/aciclovir

(b) How would you test the function of the nerve involved in Bell's palsy?
Select the correct options from the list below.

 • Ask the patient to look upwards and downwards

 • Ask the patient to look left to right

 • Ask the patient to close their eyes

 • Ask the patient to smile

 • Ask the patient to stick their tongue out

 • Ask the patient to purse their lips

 • Ask the patient to wrinkle their forehead

 • Shine a light into the patient's eye to assess their pupillary
   response

 • Check if the patient can detect sharp/blunt sensation in various
   positions all over the skin of their face

(c) Why is it important to recognise this condition early?

## Answer 3.12

(a) Bell's palsy is paralysis of the *facial* nerve which results in a facial palsy. It may be caused by a *viral* infection particularly *Herpes simplex.* Treatment involves a *short* course of *prednisolone*, as well as *aciclovir.*

(b)
- Ask the patient to close their eyes
- Ask the patient to smile
- Ask the patient to purse their lips
- Ask the patient to wrinkle their forehead

(c) Early treatment may prevent permanent disability and disfigurement.

**3.13** What are the risks of undertaking elective extractions in the following patients and how can the risks be minimised?

(a) A patient who underwent radiotherapy for an oral squamous cell cancer last year

(b) A patient who underwent radiotherapy for an oral squamous cell cancer 25 years ago

(c) A patient who has haemophilia A

(d) A patient who is HIV positive

(e) A patient who has a prosthetic heart valve

(f) A patient who had a myocardial infarction 3 weeks ago

**Answer 3.13**

(a) Patients who have had radiotherapy are at risk of getting osteoradionecrosis after extractions. Therefore prevention has a big role in these patients. However, if an extraction is needed, antibiotics are usually given until the socket has healed; this may mean a course of 4 weeks or more.

(b) The effects of radiotherapy do not decrease with time; they are permanent. Hence this patient should be managed in the same way as the patient in Question 3.13 (a).

(c) Such patients have factor VIII deficiency and therefore impaired clotting times. The severity of the condition depends on the level of factor VIII activity. All patients who require an extraction should only be treated in collaboration with their haematologist. Management usually involves preoperative blood tests, followed by transfusion of the missing factor and/or desmopressin (which stimulates factor VIII production). Other agents such as E-aminocaproic acid (Amicar) and tranexamic acid (Cyklokapron) may be used along with local measures: sutures and packing the socket with a haemostatic agent. They are usually treated as inpatients to allow postoperative monitoring.

(d) In terms of cross-infection control, universal precautions should be used. With regard to the extraction, depending on the patient's CD4:CD8 count they may be more likely to get a postoperative infection. This could mean that you would give antibiotics more readily than to a fit and healthy patient.

(e) Patients who have prosthetic heart valves are at risk of infective endocarditis and so require antibiotic prophylaxis prior to treatment. They are usually taking an anticoagulant, often warfarin. If they are, the extraction should be performed only when the international normalised ratio (INR) has been checked and is within the range that the operator is happy with. The socket is usually packed with a haemostatic aid to help with haemostasis.

(f) Elective extraction should be delayed. The likelihood of repeat myocardial infarction decreases with time from the first one. (Elective surgical procedures should be delayed for 6 months following recent myocardial infarction.)

**3.14** (a) From the list below choose the space(s) or site that infection typically spreads into from the following teeth: maxillary lateral incisor, mandibular third molar, maxillary canine.

- Sublingual
- Palatal area
- Submandibular
- Buccal
- Submasseteric
- Lateral pharyngeal
- Retropharyngeal
- Infraorbital area

(b) What are the boundaries of the submandibular space?

(c) What are the principles of management of a patient with a dental infection?

**Answer 3.14**

(a) Buccal, sublingual, submandibular, buccal, sub-masseteric, lateral pharyngeal, retropharyngeal, palatal

(b)  • Laterally: mandible below mylohyoid line

 • Medially: mylohyoid muscle

 • Inferiorly: deep cervical fascia and overlying platysma and skin

(c) Identification and removal of the cause of the infection. Steps are:

 1  Establish drainage of the abscess (intraoral/extraoral).

 2  Commence appropriate antimicrobial treatment.

 3  Assess if there is any predisposing factors for infection, eg immunosuppression, diabetes, steroid therapy.

 4  Supportive measures, analgesics, fluids, soft diet, etc.

**3.15** (a) What do you understand by the TMN classification system and what is it used for?

(b) If a patient with an intraoral tumour is staged as T2 N1 M0 what does it mean?

(c) What does Mx mean?

(d) Lesions may be treated by using a graft or a flap – what do you understand by these terms?

## Answer 3.15

(a) It is a classification system for tumours and the letters stand for:

- T – tumour
- N – nodes
- M – metastases

It is used to stage tumours.

(b) The patient had a tumour 2–4 cm in size, with a single ipsilateral lymph node less than 3 cm in diameter and no metastases. This patient has stage III disease.

(c) Distant metastases cannot be assessed.

(d) A graft is a piece of tissue that is transferred by complete separation and gains a new blood supply by ingrowth of new blood vessels. A flap has its own blood supply. They can be 'pedicled', ie their original blood supply is used, or 'free', ie they have to be 'replumbed' into the blood supply at the recipient site.

# 4
# Oral Medicine

**4.1** (a) List four possible aetiological factors for recurrent aphthae.

(b) What types of recurrent aphthae are there? How do you differentiate between the types? (eg size, location, number)

(c) How may recurrent aphthae be treated?

**Answer 4.1**

(a) Any four of the following:
- Genetic predisposition
- Immunological abnormalities
- Haematological deficiencies
- Stress
- Hormonal changes
- Gastrointestinal disorders
- Infections

(b) Minor aphthae may occur singly or in crops and they affect the non-keratinised and mobile mucosa. They are usually less than 4 mm diameter. Major aphthae usually occur as single ulcers, which may be greater than 1 cm in diameter. The masticatory mucosa and dorsum of tongue are often affected. Herpetiform aphthae usually occur in crops of ulcers which are 1–2 mm in diameter, although they may coalesce to form larger ulcers. They occur on non-keratinised mucosa.

(c) Treatment options:
- Treat underlying systemic disease
- Benzydamine (Difflam) mouthwash
- Corticosteroids (Corlan pellets, Betnesol mouthwash)
- Tetracycline mouthwashes
- Chlorhexidine mouthwash

**4.2** (a) What is angular cheilitis (stomatitis)?

(b) How does angular cheilitis differ from actinic cheilitis?

(c) List three predisposing factors for angular cheilitis.

(d) Which organisms commonly cause angular cheilitis?

(e) What medicaments could be used to treat this?

### Answer 4.2

(a) Inflammation of the skin and the labial mucous membrane at the commissures of the lips.

(b) Actinic cheilitis is a premalignant condition in which keratosis of the lip is caused by ultraviolet radiation from sunlight.

(c) Any three of the following:
- Wearing dentures and having denture-related stomatitis.
- Nutritional deficiencies, eg iron deficiency
- Immunocompromised
- Decreased vertical dimension resulting in infolding of the tissues at the corner of the mouth allowing the skin to become macerated.

(d) *Staphylococcus aureus* and *Candida albicans*

(e) Fusidic acid cream and miconazole gel

**4.3** (a) Acute pseudomembranous candidiasis or thrush is a presentation of candidal infection in the mouth. List four other ways in which candidal infections may present to a dentist?

(b) What does acute pseudomembranous candidiasis look like in the mouth?

(c) Smears are often taken from acute pseudomembranous candidiasis. How are these smears treated and what do they show?

(d) Name two azole-type drugs and two other drugs, which are not azoles, that are used to treat candidal infections.

**Answer 4.3**

(a) Any four of the following:
  - Acute atrophic candidiasis
  - Chronic atrophic candidiasis
  - Chronic erythematous candidiasis
  - Chronic hyperplastic candidiasis
  - Chronic mucocutaneous candidiasis
  - Angular stomatitis
  - Median rhomboid glossitis

(b) Whitish-yellow plaques or flecks cover the mucosa, but they can be wiped off, leaving erythematous mucosa underneath.

(c) Smears are Gram-stained and show a tangled mass of Gram-positive fungal hyphae as well as leucocytes and epithelial cells.

(d) Drugs used to treat candidal infections:
  - Azoles – any two of: ketoconazole, miconazole, fluconazole, itraconazole
  - Others – nystatin, amphotericin

**4.4** (a) Name the common types of white patches and what may cause them.

(b) What would you call a white patch that cannot be characterised clinically or pathologically as any other disease and which is not associated with any physical or chemical causative agent except the use of tobacco?

(c) What are the clinical features of the different types of white patch referred to in Question 4.4 (b)?

(d) A biopsy is usually done for these lesions. What type(s) of biopsy would be appropriate?

(e) How are these lesions treated?

**Answer 4.4**

(a) Common white patches and their causes:
- Frictional keratosis – friction
- Leukoedema – a variation of normal
- Candidal infection – *Candida albicans* infection
- Cheek biting – trauma from cheek biting
- Fordyce spots/granules – developmental (sebaceous glands in the mucosa)
- Lichen planus – unknown (lichen planus from graft versus host disease is uncommon)
- Lichenoid reactions – gold/antimalarials/dental amalgam
- Skin grafts – previous free flap to transfer tissue to cover an intraoral defect

(b) Leukoplakia

(c) Types of leukoplakia:
- Homogeneous leukoplakias
- Nodular leukoplakias
- Speckled leukoplakias

(d) Incisional and brush biopsy

(e) Treatment options for leukoplakia:
- Removal of causative agent (smoking)
- Surgical removal (traditional surgical techniques or with a laser)
- Photodynamic therapy
- Retinoids
- Specialist referral
- Regular review and biopsy as appropriate

**4.5** (a) Sjögren's syndrome is a well-known cause of a dry mouth. Name four other causes of dry mouth.

(b) What is the difference between primary and secondary Sjögren's syndrome?

(c) What type of biopsy is often carried out to diagnose Sjögren's syndrome and why?

(d) What microscopic features would the biopsy show if the patient had Sjögren's syndrome?

(e) What other investigations could be carried out to diagnose Sjögren's syndrome?

**Answer 4.5**

(a) Any four of the following:
  - Radiotherapy in the region of the salivary glands
  - Diabetes
  - Dehydration
  - Mumps
  - HIV infection
  - Anxiety states
  - Diuretics
  - Sarcoidosis
  - Amyloidosis
  - Drugs (eg antimuscarinics, antihistamines, antidepressants)

(b) Primary Sjögren's syndrome comprises dry mouth and dry eyes. In secondary Sjögren's syndrome there is dry mouth and dry eyes in association with a connective tissue disease eg rheumatoid arthritis, systemic lupus erythematosus.

(c) Labial salivary gland biopsy. This is because the minor glands are usually involved at a microscopic level even though they may not be enlarged.

(d) Focal collections of lymphoid cells are seen adjacent to blood vessels, and the greater the number of foci the worse the disease. There is also acinar atrophy.

(e) Investigations for Sjögren's syndrome:
  - Blood tests – antinuclear antibodies SSA, SSB; rheumatoid factor; erythrocyte sedimentation rate
  - Parotid salivary flow rate
  - Schirmer test
  - Sialography

**4.6** The following diseases/conditions may have signs and symptoms that are seen in and around the mouth. Match the disease/condition with the oral signs and symptoms.

| Acute leukaemia | Moon molars |
| --- | --- |
| AIDS | Fissured tongue |
| Rheumatoid arthritis | Multiple odontogenic keratocystic tumours |
| HIV carrier | Multiple supernumerary teeth |
| Melkersson–Rosenthal syndrome | Hairy leukoplakia |
| Peutz–Jeghers syndrome | Perioral pigmentation |
| Gorlin–Goltz syndrome | Koplik spots |
| Crohn's disease | Recently developed anterior open bite |
| Measles | Kaposi sarcoma |
| Marfan's syndrome | Gingival hypertrophy and bleeding |
| Syphilis | High-arched palate |
| Cleidocranial dysostosis | Wickham striae |
| Lichen planus | Cobblestoned buccal mucosa |

## Answer 4.6

| | |
|---|---|
| **Acute leukaemia** | Gingival hypertrophy and bleeding |
| **AIDS** | Kaposi sarcoma |
| **Rheumatoid arthritis** | Recently developed anterior open bite |
| **HIV carrier** | Hairy leukoplakia |
| **Melkersson–Rosenthal syndrome** | Fissured tongue |
| **Peutz–Jeghers syndrome** | Perioral pigmentation |
| **Gorlin–Goltz syndrome** | Multiple odontogenic keratocystic tumours |
| **Crohn's disease** | Cobblestoned buccal mucosa |
| **Measles** | Koplik spots |
| **Marfan syndrome** | High-arched palate |
| **Syphilis** | Moon molars |
| **Cleidocranial dysostosis** | Multiple supernumerary teeth |
| **Lichen planus** | Wickham striae |

**4.7** (a) What do you understand by the term 'erythroplasia?'

(b) What is often seen histologically?

(c) Put the following lesions in order of malignant potential with the most malignant first.

- White sponge naevus
- Erythroplasia
- Leukoplakia
- Speckled leukoplakia

(d) In the following conditions coloured lesions may appear in the mouth. What colour are they and are they localised or generalised?

- Kaposi sarcoma
- Haemangioma
- Amalgam tattoo
- Addison disease
- Irradiation mucositis

**Answer 4.7**

(a) Erythroplasia is any lesion of the oral mucosa that presents as a red velvety plaque, which cannot be characterised clinically or pathologically as any other condition.

(b) The lesions often show dysplasia or even carcinoma in situ or frank carcinoma histologically.

(c) Erythroplasia > speckled leukoplakia > leukoplakia > white sponge naevus

(d)  • Kaposi sarcoma – reddish purplish (localised)

   • Irradiation mucositis – red (generalised in region of irradiation)

   • Amalgam tattoo – blue/black (localised)

   • Haemangioma – red/purple (localised to area of haemangioma)

   • Addison disease – brown patches (localised to certain areas, eg occlusal line)

**4.8** (a) A 45-year-old patient presents with a lump in the palate. Give four possible diagnoses.

(b) List four factors in the history that may help with the diagnosis.

(c) Give four clinical features that may help you decide on the diagnosis.

(d) What investigations may be used to aid the diagnosis?

## Answer 4.8

(a) Any four of the following:
- Torus palatinus
- Unerupted tooth
- Dental abscess
- Papilloma
- Neoplasm (benign/ malignant) – salivary (pleomorphic adenoma/ adenocarcinoma); squamous cell carcinoma; lymphoma

(b) Any four of the following:
- Duration of the lump
- Associated features, eg tooth ache/periodontally involved teeth
- Any change in size/consistency.
- Any exacerbating factors, eg loose denture, denture granuloma, trauma
- Any medical conditions which may be associated with the lump, eg neurofibromatosis, drugs, hormonal, other malignancies

(c) Any four of the following:
- Position of the lump (eg in the midline – developmental torus palatinus)
- Consistency (fluid – pus/blood/cystic fluid; soft, firm, hard – tumour; bony hard – tooth, torus palatinus)
- Colour (eg red – vascular lesion or Kaposi sarcoma)
- Discharge (pus/blood/cystic fluid)
- Surface texture (uniform/ nodular or ulcerated may indicated tumour; anemone-like – papilloma)
- Associated features (eg carious upper first molar)

(d) Investigations:
- Imaging (plain radiography: panoramic radiograph, upper standard occlusal, long cone periapical)
- Computed tomography
- Biopsy (fine needle aspiration; incisional/punch biopsy; excisional)
- Blood test if suspicion of underlying blood dyscrasia

**4.9** (a) List eight features that one needs to determine in a patient presenting with pain.

(b) Which features would make you think a patient had atypical facial pain?

(c) What treatment is there for atypical facial pain?

## Answer 4.9

(a) Any eight of the following:
- Type/character of the pain
- Onset
- Duration of each episode
- Periodicity
- Site
- Radiation
- Severity
- Exacerbating and relieving factors
- Associated factors
- Previous treatment
- Effect on sleep

(b) Features of atypical facial pain:
- Pain unrelated to the anatomical divisions of nerves, and often crossing the midline
- No organic cause can be found
- Investigations do not show anything abnormal
- Long-standing and continuous, often with no exacerbating or relieving factors
- Conventional analgesics provide no relief
- Often described as unbearable

(c) Atypical facial pain is usually managed medically. The drugs of choice include tricyclic antidepressants, eg nortriptyline, amitriptyline, doxepin, trazodone, dosulepin, fluoxetine.

**4.10** (a) A 30-year-old man presents with weakness on the left side of his face. Name two possible intracranial and two possible extracranial causes.

(b) How will you tell whether a nerve lesion causing a facial weakness had an upper motor neurone cause or a lower motor neurone cause?

(c) What is Ramsay–Hunt syndrome?

(d) What treatment is indicated?

## Answer 4.10

(a) Extracranial – any two of the following:

- Bell's palsy

- Malignant parotid neoplasm

- Post-parotidectomy

- Sarcoidosis (Heerfordt syndrome)

- Incorrect administration of local anaesthetic

- Melkersson–Rosenthal syndrome

Intracranial – any two of the following:

- Cerebrovascular accident (strokes)

- Intracranial tumour

- Multiple sclerosis

- HIV

- Lyme disease

- Ramsey–Hunt syndrome

- Trauma to base of skull

(b) In a lower motor neurone lesion, the patient cannot wrinkle their forehead on the affected side, but in an upper motor neurone lesion they retain movement of their forehead. Hence to determine which one it is, you need to ask the patient to raise their eyebrows and wrinkle their forehead.

(c) Herpes zoster infection of the geniculate ganglion which produces a facial palsy. There will also be vesicles in the region of the external auditory meatus and the palate due to the viral infection.

(d) Aciclovir.

**4.11** Fill in the blanks in this paragraph on herpes zoster. The words in brackets will give you a clue.

Herpes zoster is caused by the ..................... (organism) which lies latent in ...................... . It tends to affect ..................... (age) patients. The chief complaint is ..................... . The lesions are in the form of ......................... . The treatment is ....................... at a dose of ......................... mg five times a day for ..................... . Medication for pain relief is also prescribed and ..................... (another drug) may also help with the pain and speed healing. Postherpetic neuralgia is ....................... and persisting for more than ........... ............ months.

**Answer 4.11**

Herpes zoster is caused by the *varicella zoster virus* which lies latent in *dorsal root ganglia*. It tends to affect *middle age or older* patients. The main complaint is *pain or tenderness in dermatomes*. The lesions are in the form of *rash, vesicles or ulcerations*. The treatment is *systemic aciclovir* at dose of *200–800* mg five times a day for *7 days*. Medication for pain relief] is also prescribed and *systemic corticosteroids* may also help with the pain and speed healing. Postherpetic neuralgia is *pain developing during the acute phase of herpes zoster* and persisting for more than *6* months.

**4.12** (a) Give four causes of localised gingival swelling(s).

(b) For the above four causes, which features and/or what additional investigation would aid the diagnosis.

## Answer 4.12

(a) Any four of the following:
- Periodontal abscess
- Fibrous epulis
- Denture-induced granuloma
- Pregnancy epulis
- Papilloma
- Giant cell lesion/epulis
- Tumour

(b) See according to what you have chosen from the above list:
- Periodontal abscess – associated with deep periodontal pocket and/or non-vital tooth.
- Fibrous epulis – firm, pink/red may be associated with poor oral hygiene, an excisional biopsy.
- Denture-induced granuloma – excisional biopsy and treat the cause, ie poorly fitting denture.
- Pregnancy epulis – red lesion associated with pregnancy gingivitis, excised post partum if still present.
- Papilloma – white cauliflower-like lesion, excisional biopsy.
- Giant cell lesion/epulis – purple–red lesion, radiograph, excisional biopsy and curettage, blood test to exclude central giant cell granuloma and hyperparathyroidism.
- Tumour – urgent referral to surgeon for incisional biopsy, radiography to look for bony involvement and computed tomography (CT) and magnetic resonance imaging (MRI) to stage the disease.

**4.13** (a) What are the signs and symptoms of primary herpetic gingivostomatitis?

(b) What is the causative agent?

(c) How would you treat it?

(d) Primary herpetic stomatitis may be followed by recurrent herpes labialis. How does this happen?

(e) Describe the lesions of herpes labialis and how you would manage them.

## Answer 4.13

(a) Patients have multiple vesicles in their mouth, which burst to leave painful ulcers. There is often gingivitis. Patients feel generally unwell with fever and malaise. There is cervical lymphadenopathy.

(b) Herpes simplex virus (DNA virus)

(c) Treatment of primary herpetic gingivostomatitis:
   - Bed rest, soft diet, fluids, analgesics.
   - Chlorhexidine or tetracycline mouthwash to prevent secondary infection of the ulcers.
   - Aciclovir in severe cases or medically compromised patients.

(d) The virus remains dormant in the trigeminal ganglion and can be reactivated by factors such as sunlight, stress, menstruation, immunosuppression, common cold or fever.

(e) Lesions appear at the mucocutaneous junction of the lips. The patient often has a prodromal itching/prickling sensation prior to the appearance of the lesion, which starts off as a papule and then forms vesicles that burst leaving a scab. They usually heal without scarring after 7–10 days.

   The lesions will heal without treatment but if given early, ie in the prodromal phase, antiviral cream such as penciclovir or aciclovir may prevent lesions from occurring or at least speed the healing.

**4.14**    Select from the list the most appropriate diagnostic test for the various conditions/diseases. Each option may be used only once.

| | |
|---|---|
| **Full blood count** | Sjögren syndrome |
| **History and clinical examination** | Dental abscess causing submandibular space infection |
| **Lower standard occlusal radiograph** | Benign mucous membrane pemphigoid |
| **Autoantibody blood tests** | Burning mouth |
| **Immunohistochemistry** | Glandular fever |
| **Serum angiotensin converting enzyme** | Giant cell arteritis |
| **Erythrocyte sedimentation rate** | Acute pseudomembranous candidiasis |
| **Paul Bunnell test** | Sarcoidosis |
| **Culture and sensitivity** | Trigeminal neuralgia |
| **Smear** | Submandibular duct salivary calculus |

## Answer 4.14

| | |
|---|---|
| **Sjögren syndrome** | Autoantibody blood tests |
| **Dental abscess causing submandibular space infection** | Culture and sensitivity |
| **Benign mucous membrane pemphigoid** | Immunohistochemistry |
| **Burning mouth** | Full blood count |
| **Glandular fever** | Paul Bunnell test |
| **Giant cell arteritis** | Erythrocyte sedimentation rate |
| **Acute pseudomembranous candidiasis** | Smear |
| **Sarcoidosis** | Serum angiotensin-converting enzyme |
| **Trigeminal neuralgia** | History and clinical examination |
| **Submandibular duct salivary calculus** | Lower standard occlusal radiograph |

**4.15** (a) The picture shows the buccal mucosa of a 45-year-old woman. What is the name of this common condition?

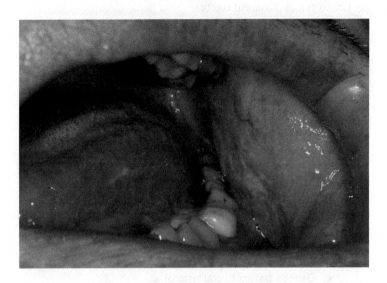

(b) This condition may have other presentations in the mouth. Name four.

(c) Where else may the patient get lesions in the mouth?

(d) In which extraoral sites may such lesions occur and what are they like?

(e) This condition may be caused by certain drugs. Name three such drugs.

## Answer 4.15

(a) Lichen planus /lichenoid reaction

(b) Any four of the following:
- Reticular (as in the picture in Question 4.15 (a))
- Atrophic
- Desquamative gingivitis
- Erosive
- Papular
- Plaque-like

(c) Dorsum of tongue and gingiva

(d) Extraoral sites:
- Flexor surfaces of wrists (purplish, papular, itchy)
- Genitals (similar to oral lesions)
- Nails (ridges)
- Head (alopecia)

(e) Any three of the following:
- β-Blockers
- Oral hypoglycaemics
- NSAIDs (non-steroidal anti-inflammatory drugs)
- Gold
- Penicillamine
- Some tricyclic antidepressants
- Antimalarials
- Thiazide diuretics
- Allopurinol

**4.16** Fill in the blanks using words from the list below. Each word can only be used once.

............... disease is due to sensitivity to .................. . Patients may suffer from malabsorption of .................., ................... and ................., and may have the following oral signs: ..............., ................ and ................. . ................. disease is a chronic .............. that may affect any part of the gastrointestinal tract, but most commonly affects the ................. . Oral signs may be seen such as mucosal tags, ...................., ..................... and ................... .

1    Crohn's/irritable bowel syndrome/coeliac disease/granulomatous disease/ulcerative colitis

2    Gluten/vitamin $B_{12}$/folate/iron/vitamin C/vitamin D

3    Cobblestone mucosa/lip swelling/oral ulceration/lichen planus/ angular cheilitis/glossitis/gingival swellings/

4    Ileum/jejunum/stomach

## Answer 4.16

*Coeliac* disease is due to sensitivity to *gluten.* Patients may suffer from malabsorption of *vitamin B$_{12}$, folate* and *iron,* and may have the following oral signs: *oral ulceration, angular cheilitis* and *glossitis. Crohn's* disease is a chronic *granulomatous* disease that may affect any part of the gastrointestinal tract, but most commonly affects the *ileum.* Oral signs may be seen such as mucosal tags, *cobblestone mucosa, lip swelling* and *oral ulceration.*

# 5
# Oral Pathology

**5.1** (a) Which of the following are histopathological features of epithelial dysplasia?

- Drop-shaped rete ridges
- Nuclear hypochromatism
- Decreased mitotic activity
- Loss of intercellular adherence
- Loss of differentiation
- Saw tooth rete ridges
- Nuclear pleomorphism
- Civatte bodies
- Loss of polarity of cells

(b) What is the difference between epithelial dysplasia, carcinoma in situ and carcinoma?

(c) What is the commonest cancer of the oral cavity?

(d) Give three risk factors for this oral cancer.

(e) If a patient has a suspicious looking ulcer on the lateral border of their tongue what type of biopsy would be carried out to aid diagnosis and why, and what should be included in the biopsy?

**Answer 5.1**

(a) Histopathological features of epithelial dysplasia:
- Drop shaped rete ridges
- Loss of intercellular adherence
- Loss of differentiation
- Nuclear pleomorphism

(b) Epithelial dysplasia is usually graded histologically as mild, moderate and severe. The term carcinoma in situ is often used to describe severe dysplasia in which the changes are seen in all the layers of the epithelium. However, the changes are confined to the epithelium in dysplasia and carcinoma in situ, whereas in carcinoma the changes are seen to extend through the basement membrane into the underlying connective tissue.

(c) Squamous cell carcinoma

(d) Any three of the following:
- Alcohol
- Tobacco
- Betel nut chewing
- Human papilloma virus
- Syphilis
- Chronic candidal infection

(e) Incisional biopsy. This should include some normal surrounding tissue and a representative portion of the lesion. Incisional biopsies are preferred so that some of the lesion is left to aid the surgeon (who may not have performed the biopsy) should they need to completely remove the lesion at a later date.

**5.2**  (a) From the options below select the correct options describing giant
cell granulomas

- They occur most commonly in the first to third decades/fourth to
  fifth decades/sixth decade plus.

- They are more common in males than females/females than
  males.

- They affect the maxilla/mandible most commonly.

- They occur anteriorly/posteriorly most commonly.

(b) Name three pathological features that you might see in a giant cell
granuloma.

(c) Why would you do blood tests for a patient with a giant cell
granuloma?

(d) What two blood tests would you do and why?

(e) Name two other non-odontogenic benign tumours of bone that affect
the jaws.

## Answer 5.2

(a) Regarding giant cell granulomas:
- They occur most commonly in the *first to third decades*.
- They are more common in *females than males*.
- They affect the *mandible* most commonly.
- They occur *anteriorly* most commonly.

(b) Any three of the following:
- Giant cells (osteoclasts)
- Vascular stroma/connective tissue
- Spindle shaped cells
- Haemosiderin (evidence of bleeding)
- Fibroblasts and evidence of collagen formation
- Osteoid

(c) Pathologically giant cell granulomas are identical to brown tumours of hyperparathyroidism. Blood tests help to distinguish between the two conditions. The blood chemistry is normal in giant cell granuloma but altered in hyperparathyroidism.

(d) Any two of the following:
- Plasma calcium levels – raised in hyperparathyroidism, normal in giant cell granuloma
- Alkaline phosphatase levels – lowered in hyperparathyroidism, normal in giant cell granuloma
- Plasma phosphate levels – lowered in hyperparathyroidism, normal in giant cell granuloma
- Parathyroid hormone levels – raised in hyperparathyroidism, normal in giant cell granuloma

(e) Any two of the following:
- Osteoma
- Osteochondroma
- Melanotic neuroectodermal tumour

**5.3** (a) What is the definition of a cyst?

(b) Are the following lesions inflammatory/developmental/non-epithelial/ neoplasm:

- Keratocystic odontogenic tumours (odontogenic keratocysts)
- Dentigerous cysts
- Radicular cysts
- Aneurysmal bone cyst

(c) From what are dentigerous cysts thought to arise and why?

(d) Where do dentigerous cysts occur most commonly?

(e) Describe what the lining and capsule of a dentigerous cyst would look like histologically.

## Answer 5.3

(a) A cyst is a pathological cavity, not formed by the accumulation of pus, with fluid, semifluid or gaseous contents, and lined by epithelium.

(b) Type of lesion:

- Keratocystic odontogenic tumours (odontogenic keratocyst) – developmental/neoplasm

- Dentigerous cysts – developmental

- Radicular cysts – inflammatory

- Aneurysmal bone cyst – non-epithelial

According to the World Health Organization (WHO) classification (2005) keratocystic odontogenic tumours are now classified as neoplasms, whereas previously they were thought to be developmental.

(c) Dentigerous cysts are attached to an unerupted tooth in the region of the amelocemental junction and so are thought to arise from the remnants of the enamel organ. The internal enamel epithelium lies over the enamel and the external enamel epithelium forms the cyst lining.

(d) They are associated with teeth that fail to erupt and so are most commonly associated with mandibular third molars and maxillary permanent canines.

(e) The lining is a thin regular layer composed of stratified squamous epithelium, which may occasionally keratinise. The capsule is composed of collagenous fibrous tissue, which is usually free from inflammatory cells. There may be scattered nests of quiescent odontogenic epithelium

**5.4** (a) What is the difference between a potentially malignant (premalignant/epithelial precursor) lesion and a potentially malignant (premalignant) condition?

(b) What do you understand by the term leukoplakia?

(c) Put the following lesions in order with the one most likely to become malignant first:

- Leukoplakia
- Speckled leukoplakia
- Erythroplasia (erythroplakia)

(d) What malignancy would they turn into?

(e) At which intraoral sites does oral cancer occur commonly?

(f) How does this cancer spread?

(g) What factors would affect survival from oral cancer?

## Answer 5.4

(a) A premalignant lesion is a lesion in which carcinoma may develop. A premalignant condition is a condition in which there is a risk of carcinoma developing within the mouth, but not necessarily in the pre-existing lesion.

(b) A white patch or plaque that cannot be characterised clinically or pathologically as any other disease and is not associated with any physical or chemical agent except the use of tobacco. It cannot be rubbed off.

(c) Erythroplasia (erythroplakia) > speckled leukoplakia > leukoplakia

(d) Squamous cell carcinoma

(e) Common sites of oral cancer:
  • Lateral border of tongue
  • Floor of mouth
  • Retromolar area

(f) Modes of spread:
  • Direct extension into adjacent tissues
  • Metastasis to regional lymph nodes
  • Late in the disease there may be haematogenous spread

(g)
  • Delay in treatment
  • Size of tumour at presentation
  • Degree of differentiation of tumour – poorly differentiated worse than well differentiated
  • Lymph node spread
  • Distant metastases
  • Position of tumour – more posterior worse prognosis
  • Malnutrition
  • Age, worse with advancing age
  • Males have a worse prognosis compared with females

**5.5** (a) In which gland do salivary calculi occur most commonly and why?

(b) What symptoms might a patient with a salivary gland obstruction complain of?

(c) Are calculi a common cause of dry mouth?

(d) If a salivary calculus is not treated what may happen to the gland and what would it look like histologically?

(e) What do you understand by the term mucocoele. What are the types of mucocoele and how do they differ?

## Answer 5.5

(a) Submandibular salivary gland. This is because of the composition of saliva produced by this gland, and the length and anatomy of the duct.

(b) Meal time syndrome – they complain of pain and swelling in the region of the gland on seeing, smelling or tasting food. The swelling gradually subsides over time. The gland may also become infected.

(c) No

(d) The gland may become infected and the patient may develop chronic sialadenitis. There is dilatation of the ductal system, and hyperplasia of the ductal epithelium and development of squamous metaplasia. There is destruction of the acini which are replaced by fibrous tissue. Histologically, there is chronic inflammatory cell infiltration of glandular parenchyma.

(e) A mucocoele is a cyst of a salivary gland, which commonly forms in the lower lip. They can be *extravasation cysts* where the saliva leaks into the surrounding tissues forming a *cyst-like space* without an epithelial lining. Much less common are *retention cysts*, where the saliva remains within the ductal system and the duct dilates to form a cyst, which is lined by epithelium. A *ranula* is a mucocoele which arises in the floor of the mouth from the sublingual salivary gland or the submandibular gland.

**5.6** Fill in the blanks using words from the following lists.

(a) Cherubism is inherited as an .................. . It usually affects
.................. . Bilateral bony swellings are seen in the ..................
and the .................. . Histologically the lesions consist of
.................. in vascular .................. .

1 Sex-linked trait/autosomal recessive trait/autosomal dominant trait

2 Young children/young adults/middle aged

3 Tuberosities/frontal region/maxillae

4 Angles of the mandible/body of the mandible/symphysis of the mandible

5 Giant cells/Birbeck granules/Civatte bodies

6 Connective tissue/epithelium

(b) Primary hyperparathyroidism is caused by .................. or adenoma
of the .................. . This results in .................. of parathormone,
which in turn .................. the plasma .................. level by
mobilising calcium. .................. swellings of the jaws can occur.
Histologically these lesions have the characteristics of a ..................
lesion.

1 Hypoplasia/atrophy/hyperplasia

2 Pituitary/thyroid/parathyroids

3 Over-production/reduction

4 Raises/lowers/depletes

5 Calcitonin/calcium/vitamin D

6 Fibrous/cyst-like/granulomatous

7 Tuberculous/granulomatous/giant cell

(c) Paget's disease commonly affects the................... . Bone resorption and ................... are irregular and exaggerated. This can lead to ................... the foramina and cranial nerve compression. Teeth may show ................... and are often difficult to extract.

1 Young/middle aged/elderly people

2 Resorption/Replacement/Reduction

3 Widening of/narrowing of/compression of

4 Caries/external resorption/hypercementosis

(d) Osteogenesis imperfecta is also known as ................... . It is usually inherited as a(an) ................... . condition. It is due to defective synthesis of type ................... collagen. Patients may have.................. ... sclera. Bones grow to ................... length, but can be distorted by multiple fractures and result in dwarfism.

1 Brittle bone/marble bone

2 Autosomal dominant/autosomal recessive/X-linked

3 I/II/III/IV

4 Red/yellow/blue/grey

5 Normal/reduced

## Answer 5.6

(a) Cherubism is inherited as an *autosomal dominant trait*. It usually affects *young children*. Bilateral bony swellings are seen in the *maxillae* and at the *angles of the mandible*. Histologically the lesions consist of *giant cells* in vascular *connective tissue*.

(b) Primary hyperparathyroidism is caused by *hyperplasia* or adenoma of the *parathyroids*. This results in *over-production* of parathormone, which in turn *raises* the plasma *calcium* level by mobilising calcium. *Cyst-like* swellings of the jaws can occur. Histologically these lesions have the characteristics of a *giant cell* lesion.

(c) Paget's disease commonly affects *elderly people*. Bone resorption and *replacement* are irregular and exaggerated. This can lead to *narrowing of* the foramina and cranial nerve compression. Teeth may show *hypercementosis* and are often difficult to extract.

(d) Osteogenesis imperfecta is also known as *brittle bone* disease. It is usually inherited as an *autosomal dominant* condition. It is due to defective synthesis of type *I* collagen. Patients may have *blue* sclera. Bones grow to *normal* length, but can be distorted by multiple fractures and result in dwarfism.

**5.7**   (a) What do you understand by the term Nikolsky's sign?

(b) Pemphigus vulgaris and mucous membrane pemphigoid are both blistering diseases, which exhibit this sign. At what level do the blisters occur in the two conditions?

(c) Why do they occur at this level?

(d) Immunohistochemistry is often used to diagnose these conditions. What do you understand by this term? What types are there and how do they differ?

(e) Molecular biology has a role in pathological diagnosis. Name one molecular biological technique.

## Answer 5.7

(a) Nikolsky's sign is when a vesicle appears on gently stroking the mucosa or skin.

(b) In pemphigus vulgaris the blisters are intra-epithelial. In mucous membrane pemphigoid they are subepithelial.

(c) The two diseases are autoimmune conditions in which autoantibodies are produced against components of the squamous epithelium of the mucosa (and skin). In pemphigus vulgaris autoantibodies are produced against an intercellular adhesion molecule (desmoglein). This causes the keratinocytes to lose their attachment to each other and vesicles/bullae are formed within the epithelium. In mucous membrane pemphigoid autoantibodies are produced against a component of the basement membrane which results in subepithelial separation.

(d) Immunohistochemistry is a technique in which specific antigens within tissue can be visualised with a light or fluorescent microscope. An antibody is applied to a section of tissue and allowed to bind. The binding site is then visualised by a fluorescent 'tag', by means of more antibodies attaching to fluorescent tags or by means of a chemical reaction to produce a colour change. There are two types of immunohistochemistry:

- Direct immunohistochemistry – a section of the patient's tissue is placed on a slide and an antibody against the test antigen is added and allowed to bind. The binding site is then visualised by one of the means described above.

- Indirect – a section of normal tissue (not from the patient) is placed on a slide and serum from the patient is added and allowed to bind. An antibody against the suspected autoantibody in the patient's serum is allowed to bind. The binding site is then visualised by one of the means described above.

(e) Any one of the following:
- Polymerase chain reaction (PCR)

- In situ hybridisation

- Northern/Southern/Western blotting

**5.8** From the right column of the table below select the histopathological features or terms that you would expect to see in the conditions or diagnoses given in the left column. Each condition or diagnosis may have one or more than one histopathological feature.

| | |
|---|---|
| **Lichen planus** | Cholesterol clefts |
| **Radicular cysts** | Saw tooth rete ridges |
| **Herpes simplex infection** | Ballooning degeneration |
| **Pemphigus vulgaris** | Acantholysis |
| **Adenoid cystic carcinoma** | Perineural invasion |
| **Denture-induced stomatitis** | Acanthosis |
| **White sponge naevus** | Rushton bodies |
| | Gram-positive hyphae |
| | Civatte bodies |
| | Epithelial hyperplasia with basket-weave appearance |

## Answer 5.8

| Lichen planus | Saw tooth rete ridges, Civatte bodies, acanthosis |
|---|---|
| Radicular cysts | Cholesterol clefts, Rushton bodies |
| Herpes simplex infection | Ballooning degeneration |
| Pemphigus vulgaris | Acantholysis |
| Adenoid cystic carcinoma | Perineural invasion |
| Denture-induced stomatitis | Acanthosis, Gram-positive hyphae |
| White sponge naevus | Epithelial hyperplasia with basket-weave appearance |

**5.9** From the right column of the table below select the site where the lesions given in the left column are most likely to occur. Each option may only be used once.

| | |
|---|---|
| **Squamous cell carcinoma** | Palate |
| **Ranula** | Upper lip |
| **Ameloblastoma** | Lower lip |
| **Kaposi sarcoma** | Dorsum of tongue |
| **Basal cell carcinoma** | Lateral border of tongue |
| **Mucus extravasation cyst** | Angle of mandible |
| **Erythema migrans** | Parotid gland |
| **Pleomorphic adenoma** | Skin of the face |
| **Lichen planus of the skin** | Flexor surfaces of the wrists |
| | Floor of mouth |

## Answer 5.9

| | |
|---|---|
| **Squamous cell carcinoma** | Lateral border of the tongue |
| **Ranula** | Floor of the mouth |
| **Ameloblastoma** | Angle of the mandible |
| **Kaposi sarcoma** | Palate |
| **Basal cell carcinoma** | Skin of the face |
| **Mucus extravasation cyst** | Lower lip |
| **Erythema migrans** | Dorsum of the tongue |
| **Pleomorphic adenoma** | Parotid gland |
| **Lichen planus of the skin** | Flexor surfaces of the wrists |

**5.10** (a) Please select the most appropriate term/word to fill in the blanks:

Most salivary gland tumours occur in the................... gland. Most salivary gland tumours in the parotid gland are ................... . Salivary gland tumours in the ................... gland are malignant more often than those in the submandibular gland. Most salivary tumours in the sublingual gland are ................... .

1 Parotid/sublingual/submandibular

2 Benign/malignant

(b) Name one benign salivary gland tumour and three malignant salivary gland tumours.

(c) Which salivary gland tumours tend to infiltrate along nerve sheaths?

(d) What do you understand by the term necrotising sialometaplasia?

(e) Where are you likely to see this condition?

(f) What factors predispose to this condition?

## Answer 5.10

(a) • Most salivary gland tumours occur in the *parotid* gland. Most salivary gland tumours in the parotid gland are *benign*. Salivary gland tumours in the *sublingual* gland are malignant more often than those in the submandibular gland. Most salivary tumours in the sublingual gland are *malignant*.

Note: Percentage of malignant tumours: in the parotid glands – 15–32%; in the submandibular glands – 41–44%; in the sublingual glands – 70–90%; and in the minor salivary glands – 50%. (WHO 2005).

(b) Benign – any one of the following:
• Pleomorphic adenoma

• Warthin tumour

Malignant – any three of the following:
• Adenoid cystic carcinoma

• Mucoepidermoid carcinoma

• Acinic cell carcinoma

• Carcinoma in ex-pleomorphic adenoma

(c) Adenoid cystic carcinoma and polymorphous low-grade adenocarcinoma.

(d) This lesion looks clinically and histologically like a squamous cell or mucoepidermoid carcinoma but is caused by chronic inflammation of minor salivary glands often with necrosis of acini. There is squamous metaplasia of duct tissue.

(e) The palate

(f) Predisposing factors:
• Smoking

• Male

• Middle age

**5.11** (a) From which structure are odontogenic keratocystic tumours thought to arise?

(b) Why do keratocystic odontogenic tumours (odontogenic keratocysts) have a strong tendency to recur after removal?

(c) Which age group do they most commonly occur in?

(d) Which is the most common site of presentation?

(e) List four characteristic histological features of odontogenic keratocystic tumours.

(f) What syndrome are odontogenic keratocystic tumours associated with?

(g) What are the characteristic facial features in these patients?

(h) What other lesions do these patients present with in the head and neck?

## Answer 5.11

(a) Dental lamina or its remnants

(b) Reasons for recurrence:
- They are difficult to remove intact due to the thin fragile cyst lining.
- They often have 'daughter' cysts.
- They are multilocular with finger-like extensions within the bone.
- The keratocyst epithelium proliferates rapidly.
- The remnants of the dental lamina may produce more lesions.

(c) 20–30 years

(d) Angle of the mandible

(e) Any four of the following:
- Uniform thickness of epithelium
- Flat basement membrane, 5–10 cells thick
- Elongated palisaded basal cells
- Eosinophilic layer of prekeratin in parakeratinised cyst
- Orthokeratin formation and well defined granular cell layer in orthokeratinised cysts
- Folded cyst lining
- Thin fibrous wall

(f) Basal cell naevus syndrome, Gorlin–Goltz syndrome

(g) Frontal and parietal bossing, broad nasal root

(h) Multiple naevoid basal cell carcinomas

**5.12** (a) Lichen planus is a chronic inflammatory disease. Which tissues does it commonly affect?

(b) Which age group is commonly affected?

(c) Reticular lichen planus and atrophic lichen planus are common clinical presentations. Name two other clinical appearances of lichen planus.

(d) List four typical histological features of (reticular) lichen planus

(e) What other histological changes might be seen in the epithelium if the lesion were atrophic?

(f) What serious complication can arise in lichen planus?

(g) Name another connective tissue disorder that can give rise to intraoral lesions similar to lichen planus.

## Answer 5.12

(a) Skin and mucous membranes

(b) Over 40 years

(c) Any two of the following:
- Desquamative gingivitis
- Erosive
- Papular
- Plaque-like

(d) Any four of the following:
- Hyperkeratosis/parakeratosis
- Saw tooth rete ridges
- Band-like lymphoplasmacytic infiltration in the juxta-epithelial lamina propria
- Oedema extending into the basal layers resulting in liquefaction degeneration of the basal cell layer
- Lymphocyte infiltration into the basal layers of the epithelium and CD8 lymphocytes predominate
- Hyaline or Civatte bodies in epithelium

(e) There is thinning and flattening of the epithelium

(f) Malignant change

(g) Lupus erythematosus

# 6

# Oral Radiography/Radiology

**6.1** (a) What is tomography?

(b) How is this achieved?

(c) What is a focal trough?

(d) Give five indications for dental panoramic tomography.

(e) What do you understand by the term 'ghost shadows' with respect to dental panoramic tomography?

(f) What would an air shadow look like on a dental panoramic tomograph and why do they take on this appearance?

(g) What radiation dosage does a patient receive in this procedure?

## Answer 6.1

(a) It is a technique for producing images of a slice or section of an object.

(b) The X-ray tube and the film cassette carrier are connected and move synchronously but in opposite directions about a pivoting point. The pivoting point will appear in focus on the radiograph.

(c) Only a slice of the object is in focus on the tomograph and this is called the focal trough.

(d) Any five of the following:
- Assessment of third molars.
- Assessment for fractures of the mandible.
- To assess bone heights in periodontal disease with pockets greater than 5 mm in depth.
- Orthodontic assessment.
- To assess bony lesions of the mandible and maxilla.
- Implant planning.
- To assess bony disorders of the temporomandibular joints.
- To assess antral disease.

(e) Ghost shadows are shadows cast by anatomical structures such as the cervical vertebrae and the mandible and palate, which are outside the focal trough on the panoramic radiograph. They appear on the opposite side of the real image counterpart and slightly higher up than the real image.

(f) Air shadows are radiolucent because there is no photon absorption wheras there is in tissue.

(g) 0.007–0.026 mSv depending on how the radiograph is taken.

**6.2** (a) Name the error that could have occurred to produce the following faults in a panoramic radiograph.

(i) The film shows anterior teeth that are out of focus and magnified.

(ii) The molars are larger on one side than the other.

(iii) There is vertical or horizontal distortion of one part of the image.

(iv) The radiograph is too dark.

(b) What do you understand by the terms development and fixation with regard to radiographs?

**Answer 6.2**

(a) Errors producing the faults given in the question are:

(i) The patient is positioned too far from the film.

(ii) The patient has their head to one side or the other so they are asymmetrically positioned in the machine.

(iii) The patient has moved while the radiograph was being taken.

(iv) There are several reasons:

- Overexposure – due to increased exposure time either by operator error or faulty equipment.

- Overdevelopment – due to excessive time in the developer solution, the solution being too warm or too concentrated.

- Fogging – due to poor storage of the film or light leaking onto film during development.

- Patient with very thin tissues.

(b) Development is when the sensitised silver halide crystals in the film emulsion are converted to metallic silver, which is black in colour and produces the black/grey part of the image. Fixation is when the unsensitised silver halide crystals on the film emulsion are removed. This produces the white/transparent part of the image.

**6.3** (a) How often must a dentist attend a radiation protection update course?

(b) List five methods you could use to minimise the radiation dose to a patient having an intraoral radiograph.

(c) What do you understand by the term somatic stochastic effects of ionising radiation? What is the safe dose of ionising radiation to prevent these effects?

(d) How does ionising radiation damage the body?

(e) What is the estimated risk of developing fatal cancer from dental panoramic radiography?

### Answer 6.3

(a) Five hours of radiation protection training every five years as part of continuing professional development.

(b) Any five of the following:
- Justification

- High-speed film

- Rectangular collimation

- Quality control

- Optimal kV (70 kV)

- Digital radiography

(c) Stochastic means governed by the laws of probability or random. Hence stochastic effects are effects that may develop. There is no safe dose as they might occur after any dose of ionising radiation so every exposure carries the risk of stochastic effects. Obviously the lower the ionising radiation dose the lower the likelihood of damage, although the amount of damage is not related to the size of the inducing dose.

(d) The effects can cause direct or indirect damage. Direct damage involves ionising biological molecules, eg point mutations in DNA. Indirect damage occurs from ionising water, which leads to the formation of free radicals. These may combine to form highly reactive species which cause damage.

(e) 1:2 000 000

**6.4** (a) From the right column of the table below select the most appropriate image to show the structures and conditions in the left column. Each option may be used once or not at all.

| | |
|---|---|
| **A fractured zygomatic arch** | Mandibular standard occlusal radiograph |
| **Periodontal pocketing around lower incisors** | Bitewing radiographs |
| **Interproximal caries** | 10° occipitomental radiograph |
| **Internal derangement of the temporomandibular joint** | CT scan of the face |
| **An impacted lower third molar** | Long cone periapical radiographs |
| **A fluid level in the maxillary antrum** | Bisecting angle periapical radiographs |
| **A blow-out fracture of the orbital floor** | MRI scan |
| **A salivary calculus in the submandibular duct** | Submentovertex radiograph |
| **Presence of an impacted permanent upper canine** | Maxillary standard occlusal radiograph |
| | Panoramic radiograph |
| | Reverse Townes radiograph |

## Answer 6.4

| | |
|---|---|
| **A fractured zygomatic arch** | Submentovertex radiograph |
| **Periodontal pocketing around lower incisors** | Long cone periapical radiographs |
| **Interproximal caries** | Bitewing radiographs |
| **Internal derangement of the temporomandibular joint** | MRI scan |
| **An impacted lower third molar** | Panoramic radiograph |
| **A fluid level in the maxillary antrum** | 10° occipitomental radiograph |
| **A blow-out fracture of the orbital floor** | CT scan of the face |
| **A salivary calculus in the submandibular duct** | Mandibular standard occlusal radiograph |
| **Presence of an impacted permanent upper canine** | Maxillary standard occlusal radiograph |

**6.5** (a) What do you understand by the ALARP principle.

(b) List seven factors that can help achieve this principle.

(c) Should lead aprons be used routinely in dental radiography? Please give a reason for your answer.

(d) What are the annual dose limits of radiation for non-classified workers?

### Answer 6.5

(a) ALARP an acronym that stands for 'as low as reasonably practicable' and is meant to minimise exposure to radiation.

(b) Any seven of the following:
- Every radiograph must be justified.
- All exposures should be kept as low as reasonably practicable – they should be optimised.
- There should be limitation of radiation dose.
- There should be written guidelines for exposure setting for radiographs.
- The fastest speed film should be used that will give a good quality image (usually E).
- A rectangular collimator should be used.
- There should be minimal skin to focus distances (> 60 kV = 20 cm).
- Film holders should be used rather than patients holding the film.
- When referring a patient the radiographs should be sent with the patient to avoid further radiation.
- All radiographs should be evaluated and an entry made in the patient's notes.
- There should be a quality assurance programme in place to optimise results.

(c) There is no justification for the routine use of lead aprons in dental radiography as reducing radiation is best achieved by implementing measures such as clinical judgement, equipment optimisation and radiographic technique. This is given in the 'Guidance Notes for Dental Practitioners on the Safe Use of X-ray Equipment' published in 2001 by the Department of Health.

(d) 6 mSv

**6.6** (a) What is sialography? Give two indications and contraindications for using it.

(b) Submandibular duct salivary calculi/obstructions can sometimes be seen on routine radiography. On which radiographic views would you see submandibular duct salivary calculi?

(c) Ultrasound can be used for imaging salivary glands. Give four advantages of using ultrasound for this purpose.

**Answer 6.6**

(a) Sialography involves introducing a radiopaque medium into the ductal system of a major salivary gland and then taking a radiographic image.

Indications:
- Obstructions in the ductal system, eg calculi.

- It is used to assess the structure of the gland and ductal system and to see if there is any destruction or changes in them.

Contraindications – any two of the following:
- Allergy to iodine-containing compounds.

- Infection in the gland.

- A calculus close to the duct orifice which may be pushed further back by the introduction of contrast medium.

(b) Dental panoramic radiograph and lower standard occlusal

(c) Any four of the following:
- No ionising radiation used.

- Excellent for superficial masses.

- Can use it to guide fine needle aspiration.

- Can use to differentiate between solid and cystic masses.

- It can identify radiolucent calculi not seen on radiographs.

- It can be used to break up calculi by lithotripsy.

- Intraoral masses can be visualised with small probes.

**6.7** (a) Describe what a keratocystic odontogenic tumour (odontogenic keratocyst) may look like on a radiograph.

(b) Describe what a dentigerous cyst may look like on a radiograph.

(c) If a patient had a lesion at the angle of their mandible what radiographic views could be taken to demonstrate it and what would each view show?

## Answer 6.7

(a) Radiographic features of a keratocystic odontogenic tumour:
- Radiolucent lesion
- Well defined
- Multilocular although may be unilocular
- Rounded margins
- Adjacent teeth may be displaced
- Tooth roots are not usually resorbed

(b) Radiographic features of a dentigerous cyst:
- Radiolucent lesion
- Well circumscribed
- Usually unilocular but there may be pseudo-loculation due to bony trabeculae
- Rounded
- Contains the crown of a tooth, or lies adjacent to the crown of a tooth
- Associated tooth is usually displaced

(c) A dental panoramic radiograph, sectional dental panoramic tomograph or oblique lateral views would show the lesion. The mesiodistal and superior/inferior dimensions of the lesion would be evident as well as association with any teeth, the inferior dental canal, etc. A posterior–anterior (PA) view of the mandible will show any buccolingual expansion of the mandible.

**6.8**  (a) One technique for taking periapical radiographs is the paralleling technique. Name another technique.

(b) Give an advantage of using this technique compared with the paralleling technique.

(c) What are the advantages of using a paralleling technique in periapical radiography?

(d) Describe how you would set up the tube head to take a bitewing radiograph and why.

## Answer 6.8

(a) Bisecting angle technique

(b) Any one of the following:
- Positioning of the film packet in any area of the mouth is usually more comfortable for the patient.
- It is straightforward and quick.
- The length of the crowns and roots should be the same as the teeth being radiographed if the film and tube have been correctly positioned.

(c) Advantages of using a paralleling technique:
- No image distortion.
- Images are reproducible at different visits and with different operators.
- There is no 'coning off' of the image.
- Rectangular collimation will reduce the radiation dose to patients.
- Periodontal bone levels and the crowns of teeth are well shown.
- No superimposition of the zygomatic buttress on the maxillary molars.

(d) The X-ray beam is angled downwards by 5–8° to account for the curve of Monson on the occlusal plane. It is also aimed through the contact points at right angles to the teeth and the film packet to avoid overlap of the contact areas.

**6.9** (a) When taking a radiograph a certain part of the room is designated as controlled area. What do you understand by this term?

(b) How large is this area? Give an example of the radius for a machine taking panoramic dental radiographs and intraoral periapicals.

(c) What measures are advised with regard to the above?

(d) Digital radiography is becoming more popular. What is used instead of a film packet when taking a digital radiograph?

(e) Give four advantages of digital radiography over conventional radiography.

**Answer 6.9**

(a) The controlled area is within the primary beam until it has gone far enough to be reduced in strength or gone through shielding. It also includes the area around the patient and X-ray tube.

(b) The size of the area depends on the voltage of the equipment. For an intraoral radiograph the radius is 1 m and for a panoramic radiograph it is 1.5 (as panoramic machines have a peak operating potential greater than 70 kVp).

(c) Hazard lights which should be illuminated during the exposure, and signs on the door are needed.

(d) A charged couple device (CCD), a complementary metal oxide semiconductor, a photostimulable phosphor imaging plate (PSPP)

(e) Any four of the following:
- No processing faults.
- No risk from handling the chemicals involved in processing.
- Lower radiation dose as the image receptors are more sensitive than conventional film.
- Ease of storage of images.
- Ease of transfer of images.
- Electronic enhancement of images.

**6.10**

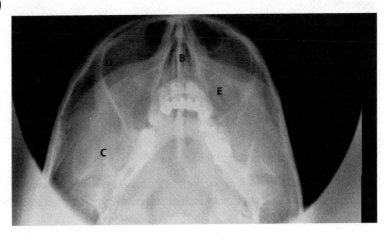

(a) What view is shown in the figure?

(b) Give four indications for taking this view.

(c) What can you see on this view?

(d) Indicate the structures labelled A–E?

**Answer 6.10**

(a) Occipito-mental view (30°)

(b) Any four of the following:
- Suspected fracture of the zygomatic complex
- Middle third facial injuries
- Le Fort I, II, III fractures
- Nasoethmoidal complex fractures
- Orbital fractures (although with the above, except for zygomatic fractures, other imaging such as computed tomography is also often done).
- Coronoid process fractures
- Frontal sinus and ethmoidal sinus visualisation

(c) Fracture of the right zygomatic complex with disruption at the inferior orbital rim and the zygomatic buttress.

(d)
- A: Frontal sinus
- B: Nasal septum
- C: Coronoid process
- D: Lateral orbital margin
- E: Maxillary antrum
- F: Sphenoidal sinus

**6.11** A 30-year-old man was injured in a road traffic accident. He was taken by ambulance to accident and emergency. On examination he had sustained head injury and a laceration. He is conscious with no focal neurological signs.

(a) What view is shown below?

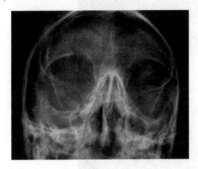

(b) What abnormality is seen on this radiograph?

(c) If you wanted more information about the orbital fracture which type of image would you order?

(d) A similar image can be used if a patient had an orbital floor fracture. What is often seen on the image?

(e) A similar radiograph is shown below. What abnormality is seen in the mandible?

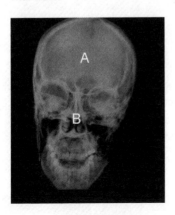

(f) Which radiographic view would give you a better view of this abnormality?

(g) What are the structures labelled A and B?

**Answer 6.11**

(a) PA view of the skull

(b) Fracture of his frontal bone/superior orbital margin

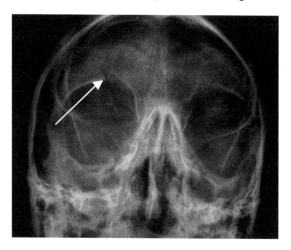

(c) A CT scan

(d) Herniation of orbital contents into the maxillary antrum.

(e) Fracture of the right angle of the mandible

(f) It would be identified better on a PA view of the jaws/mandible, a panoramic radiograph or an oblique lateral view.

(g)
  - A: Sagittal suture
  - B: Inferior turbinate

**6.12** (a) Describe what you can see on the radiograph shown in the figure.

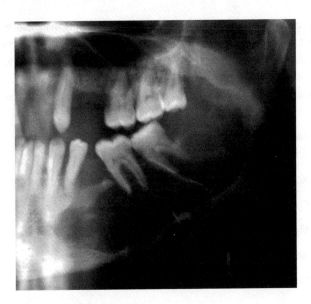

(b) What is your differential diagnosis?

(c) The inferior dental canal is seen clearly on this view. How might the inferior dental canal look on a radiograph if it was associated with an impacted wisdom tooth?

## Answer 6.12

(a) A radiolucent area at the angle and body of left side of the mandible. It extends from the first premolar to the ascending ramus of the mandible. It is multilocular with distinct septa. The outline is smooth, scalloped and well defined, and there are internal septa. There is bony expansion of the mandible and displacement of inferior dental canal. There is no resorption of the tooth roots.

(b) Differential diagnosis:
- Ameloblastoma
- Keratocystic odontogenic tumour (odontogenic keratocyst)
- Calcifying epithelial odontogenic tumour (early stage)
- Myxoma
- Ameloblastic fibroma
- Haemangioma

(c)
- Narrowing of the tramlines
- Deviation of the tramlines
- Loss of the tramlines
- Radiolucent banding across the root

# 7

# Human Disease and Therapeutics

**7.1**  (a)  What is the mechanism of action of the following autoimmune reactions? Give an example of each.

- Type I
- Type II
- Type III
- Type IV

(b)  What signs and symptoms might a patient experiencing a type I reaction show?

(c)  Latex allergy is common in the general population. Name six items in a dental surgery that contain latex.

**Answer 7.1**

(a) Mechanism of action and any one of the examples given:
- Type I – immediate reaginic (anaphylaxis, allergic asthma, allergic rhinitis)

- Type II – antibody dependent (transfusion reactions, myasthenia gravis)

- Type III – immune complex (rheumatoid arthritis, systemic lupus erythematosus)

- Type IV – cell mediated (contact dermatitis, pemphigoid, Hashimoto thyroiditis)

(b) Rash, itching, facial flushing, tingling of face, swelling of tongue, wheeze, stridor, collapse.

(c) Any six of the following:
- Dental anaesthetic cartridges (except Citanest)

- Examination and surgical gloves

- Rubber dam

- Mouth props

- Anaesthetic masks and hoses

- Blood pressure cuffs

- Orthodontic elastics

- Mixing bowls

- Endodontic stops

**7.2** (a) What type of drug is warfarin and what is its mode of action?

(b) How is warfarin treatment monitored?

(c) List three medical conditions for which patients may be prescribed warfarin.

(d) Which of the following drugs may interact with warfarin? Do they enhance or decrease the action of the warfarin?

- Fluconazole

- Penicillin

- Metronidazole

- Adrenaline

- Paracetamol

- Carbemazepine

(e) What type of drug is tranexamic acid? How is it administered and when would it be used?

### Answer 7.2

(a) Warfarin is an anticoagulant, and it is a vitamin K antagonist.

(b) By measuring a patient's INR (international normalised ratio), which is the ratio of patient's prothrombin time to control prothrombin time.

(c) Any three of the following:
- Atrial fibrillation
- Prosthetic heart valves
- Deep vein thrombosis
- Pulmonary embolus
- Cerebrovascular accident
- Antiphospholipid syndrome

(d) Drugs that interact with warfarin:
- Fluconazole – enhances anticoagulant effect
- Metronidazole – enhances anticoagulant effect
- Carbamazepine – reduces anticoagulant effect

(e) Tranexamic acid is an antifibrinolytic agent. It may be used topically as a mouthwash or by soaking swabs in it and getting the patient to bite on them. It can also be given orally or intravenously. It is used to prevent and control bleeding especially during and after the procedure.

**7.3**    What are the dental implications of the following findings in a patient's medical history:

(a) The patient is taking glyceryl trinitrate (GTN)

(b) The patient is taking Insulatard

(c) The patient is taking nifedipine

(d) The patient has had infective endocarditis in the past but is not allergic to penicillin

(e) The patient has a septal defect in their heart

(f) The patient has asthma

## Answer 7.3

(a) GTN is a vasodilator and also reduces left ventricular work by reducing venous return. Hence it is used to provide symptomatic relief in angina. Angina occurs when there is an imbalance between the demand and supply of blood to the heart and the patient experiences crushing central chest pain that can radiate down the left arm. An attack may be precipitated by dental treatment. Reducing stress by providing good anaesthesia and not subjecting patients to long appointments will minimise the likelihood of the patient having an attack. In addition, the patient should take GTN at the start of an appointment.

(b) Insulatard is an insulin preparation that is used to control the blood glucose levels in patients with insulin-dependent diabetes mellitus. Patients self-administer Insulatard subcutaneously. Diabetic patients have poor wound healing and are more susceptible to infections. Hence they are prone to gingivitis, rapidly progressing periodontal disease and oral candidal infections. They may also have xerostomia. Treatment should be timed so that it does not interfere with the meal times as hypoglycaemia may develop and the patient may collapse.

(c) Nifedipine is a calcium-channel blocker used to treat hypertension. Hypertensive patients are at increased risk of other cardiovascular disease. Routine dental treatment may need to be postponed if the patient's blood pressure is greater than 160/110 mmHg. Hypertensive patients are more likely to have excessive bleeding following extractions. Nifedipine can cause gingival hyperplasia.

(d) Patients who have had infective endocarditis require antibiotics prior to any 'blood letting' dental procedure. At present there are two sets of guidelines in use in the UK. According to the BSAC 2006 guidelines, 3g oral amoxicillin one hour pre op is adequate. However, according to the BNF (British National Formulary) 2007 guidelines, iv amoxicillin 1g and iv genatmycin 120mg at induction followed by 500mg oral amoxicillin six hours later is adequate.

(e) Patients who have septal defects are given antibiotic cover under the BNF 2007 guidelines, either 3g oral amoxicillin one hour pre op or 600mg clindamycin if they are allergic to penicillin in the previous month. According to BSAC 2007 they do not require antibiotic cover.

(f) Asthma is a condition in which there is reversible obstruction of the bronchioles, resulting in an expiratory wheeze that may progress to an inability to breathe. Asthmatic patients may have multiple allergies. Care should be taken when prescribing non-steroidal anti-inflammatory drugs (NSAIDs) as they may precipitate an asthma attack. Some patients take inhaled steroids and are at risk of candidal infections of the mouth. Some may be taking oral steroids and so are theoretically at risk of a steroid collapse during a stressful procedure. Sedation in the dental surgery should be used with great care.

**7.4** Which drug, dose and route (see opposite page) should be used in the emergencies listed below? Choose the most appropriate from the options given below. Each option may be used once, more than once or not at all.

| Emergency | Drug | Dose | Route |
|---|---|---|---|
| Anaphylaxis | | | |
| Hypoglycaemic collapse | | | |
| Status epilepticus | | | |
| Myocardial infarction | | | |
| Asthmatic attack | | | |

| Drugs | Dosage | Route |
|---|---|---|
| Adrenaline | 10 mg | Inhalational |
| Diazepam | 10 ml of 1:1000 | Intramuscular |
| Diclofenac | 1 g | Intravenous |
| Glucose | 100 mg | Oral |
| Glyceryl trinitrate | 0.5–1 ml of 1:1000 | PR |
| Insulin | 5 ml of a 50% solution | Subcutaneous |
| Nitrous oxide/ oxygen | 50 ml of a 50% solution | Sublingual |
| Salbutamol | 2 puffs/nebuliser | |

**Answer 7.4**

| Emergency | Drug | Dose | Route |
|---|---|---|---|
| Anaphylaxis | Adrenaline | 0.5–1 ml of 1:1000 | Intramuscular |
| Hypoglycaemic collapse | Glucose | 50 ml of a 50% solution | Intravenous |
| Status epilepticus | Diazepam | 10 mg | Intravenous |
| Myocardial infarction | Nitrous oxide/ oxygen, | | Inhalational |
| Asthmatic attack | Salbutamol | 2 puffs/nebuliser | Inhalational |

**7.5** (a) What do the following terms mean?

- Autograft

- Allograft

- Xenograft

(b) Give an example of each.

(c) Many patients who receive transplants are on immunosuppressant medication. What are the side-effects of immunosuppressant medication?

(d) Ciclosporin is a commonly used immunosuppressant drug. Name a complication that can occur with its use.

(e) Name another commonly used immunosuppressant drug.

## Answer 7.5

(a)
- Autograft – from the same person
- Allograft – from an individual of the same species
- Xenograft – from a different species

(b) Examples:
- Autograft – iliac crest bone to jaw
- Allograft – kidney, liver, cornea, heart, lung
- Xenograft – porcine heart valves

(c) Side-effects of immunosuppressants:
- Increased risk of infection
- Increased risk of cancer (skin and haematological)

(d) Any one of the following:
- Gingival hyperplasia
- Diabetes
- Hypertension

(e) Any one of the following:
- Azathioprine
- Mycophenolate

**7.6**   (a) What are the major systemic side-effects of steroids? List four the systems that may be affected and give two examples of each.

(b) Name an oral condition for which a patient may be prescribed topical steroids.

(c) Name a head and neck condition for which a patient may be prescribed systemic steroids.

**Answer 7.6**

(a) Any four of the following systems and any two of the following examples:
- Gastrointestinal – peptic ulceration, dyspepsia, oesophageal candidal infection

- Musculoskeletal – proximal myopathy, osteoporosis, vertebral and long bone fractures

- Endocrine – adrenal suppression, Cushing's syndrome, hirsutism, weight gain, increased appetite and increased susceptibility to infection

- Neuro-psychiatric – mood changes, depression, euphoria, psychological dependence psychosis

- Eye – glaucoma, increased intraocular pressure

- Skin – skin atrophy, telangiectasia, bruising and acne

(b) Any one of the following:
- Recurrent aphthous ulceration

- Lichen planus

(c) Any one of the following:
- Bell's palsy

- Giant cell arteritis

- Pemphigoid

- Pemphigus

- Sarcoidosis

**7.7**   (a) What causes HIV disease?

    (b) How does it spread?

    (c) What part of the immune response is affected?

    (d) Name five oral conditions/lesions strongly associated with HIV disease.

    (e) What types of drug are used to treat HIV disease?

    (f) What is the importance of HIV for a dentist?

**Answer 7.7**

(a) HIV disease is caused by infection with human immunodeficiency viruses, which are RNA retroviruses.

(b) HIV infection can be transmitted:
- Sexually
- Through blood and blood products
- Intravenous drug misuse
- From mother to child

(c) T cell mediated immunity, in particular, CD4-positive lymphocytes.

(d) Any five of the following:
- Kaposi sarcoma
- Candidal infections
- Hairy leukoplakia
- Periodontal disease (gingivitis and periodontitis)
- Non-Hodgkin lymphoma
- Necrotising ulcerative gingivitis
- Ulcers

(e) Drugs used to treat HIV disease:
- Nuclcoside reverse transcriptase inhibitors and non-nucleoside reverse transcriptase inhibitors
- Protease inhibitors

(f) There is risk of cross-infection. The patient is immunocompromised and hence may be more susceptible to infection than a healthy patient. They would be on multidrug treatment.

**7.8** (a) How is liver disease relevant to dentistry?

(b) How are the following diseases spread?
- Hepatitis A
- Hepatitis B
- Hepatitis C
- Hepatitis D

(c) What infective agent causes hepatitis B?

(d) Which type of hepatitis can people be vaccinated against?

(e) Which type of hepatitis must all dental personnel be vaccinated against?

(f) What type of vaccine is used in (e)?

## Answer 7.8

(a) Relevance of liver disease to dentistry:
- Patients with liver disease may have excess bleeding because of abnormal clotting factors.
- Patients with liver disease may be unable to metabolise drugs normally.
- Patients with liver disease may have a transmissible disease that could be a potential cross-infection risk.
- Patients may have delayed healing due to hypoproteinaemia and hence immunoglobulin deficiency.
- Administration of intravenous sedation may result in coma.

(b) Mode of spread of hepatitis:
- Hepatitis A – oro-faecal
- Hepatitis B – parental, sexually and perinatally
- Hepatitis C – parental, sexually and perinatally
- Hepatitis D – parental, sexually and perinatally

(c) A DNA virus called hepatitis B virus

(d) A and B

(e) Hepatitis B

(f) Recombinant DNA hepatitis surface antigen (HbsAg)

**7.9**  (a) Match the drug with the appropriate statement.

| | |
|---|---|
| **Aciclovir** | Inactivated by gastric acid and is best given by injections |
| **Amphotericin** | Active against many streptococci |
| **Benzyl penicllin** | Active against β-lactamase producing bacteria as it contains clavulanic acid |
| **Co-amoxiclav** | May cause pseudomembranous colitis |
| **Clindamycin** | Associated with 'red man' syndrome |
| **Metronidazole** | Active against anaerobes |
| **Phenoxymethylpenicillin** | Is a polyene antifungal drug |
| **Vancomycin** | Can be used to treat herpes simplex infections |

(b) Give four indications of systemic antibiotics in dentistry.

**Answer 7.9**

(a)

| Benzyl penicillin | Inactivated by gastric acid and is best given by injections |
|---|---|
| Phenoxymethylpenicillin | Active against many streptococci |
| Co-amoxiclav | Active against β-lactamase producing bacteria due to containing clavulanic acid |
| Clindamycin | May cause pseudomembranous colitis |
| Vancomycin | Associated with 'red man' syndrome |
| Metronidazole | Active against anaerobes |
| Amphotericin | Is a polyene antifungal drug |
| Aciclovir | Can be used to treat herpes simplex infections |

(b) Indications of systemic antibiotics in dentistry:

- Treatment of spreading infection.

- Prevention of postoperative infection.

- Antibiotic cover to prevent infective endocarditis.

- Prevention of infection following oral and maxillofacial trauma.

**7.10**  (a) What do you understand by the term anaemia?

    (b) What clinical features other than oral symptoms may the patient have?

    (c) What oral conditions may anaemia predispose to?

    (d) What is sickle cell disease?

    (e) Which group of patients is most likely to be affected?

    (f) When is it of concern to a dentist?

## Answer 7.10

(a) Anaemia is a reduction in the oxygen-carrying capacity of the blood. It is defined by a low value for haemoglobin (females < 115 g/l and males <135 g/l).

(b) Symptoms vary with severity of the anaemia and range from pallor, fatigue, weakness, breathlessness, tachycardia and palpitations, dizziness, tinnitus, vertigo, headache and dyspnoea (shortness of breath) on exertion to angina, cardiac failure and gastrointestinal disturbances.

(c) Anaemia predisposes to:
- Glossitis
- Candidal infections and angular cheilitis
- Recurrent aphthae

(d) Sickle cell disease is an autosomal recessive condition in which there is a defect in a haemoglobin chain, which can cause haemolysis and anaemia. At low oxygen tensions or acidaemia the abnormal haemoglobin (HbS) polymerises, resulting in sickling of the red blood cells and blockage of the microcirculation.

(e) People of African or African Caribbean origin are most often affected.

(f) Sickling occurs under low oxygen tensions and so sedation may cause a problem and may precipitate a crisis, hence should be avoided in general practice. General anaesthetics also have the potential to cause a sickling crisis and should only be given when absolutely necessary and following adequate preoperative assessment.

**7.11** (a) Midazolam is often used for sedation in dentistry. Name three other drugs that are used in dentistry to control anxiety.

(b) How are these drugs administered?

(c) How does midazolam work?

(d) If you were sedating a patient with midazolam in a surgery what preoperative instructions would you give them regarding the sedation?

(e) What equipment should you have in your surgery if you are planning to administer an intravenous sedative to your patient?

**Answer 7.11**

(a) Any three of the following:
- Diazepam
- Temazepam
- Nitrous oxide
- Propofol

(b) Mode of administration of sedative drugs:
- Midazolam – intravenous titration, intranasal for children
- Diazepam – oral
- Temazepam – oral
- Nitrous oxide – inhalation
- Propofol – intravenous titration

(c) By blocking the GABA (γ-amino butyric acid) receptors centrally.

(d) Preoperative instructions for midazolam sedation:
- Explanation of procedure.
- Requirement of an escort.
- Information on food intake prior to the procedure.
- Should not use machinery or drive after the procedure.
- Should not sign any legal document after the procedure.
- Should not supervise small children after the procedure.

(e) Equipment necessary for intravenous sedation:
- Pulse oximeter
- Instrument for blood pressure measurement
- Oxygen with or without Ambu bag
- Reversal agent (eg flumazenil if sedating with midazolam)
- Resuscitation equipment

Staff should also be adequately trained in the procedure.

**7.12** (a) What groups of analgesic drugs could you prescribe to a patient with dental pain? Give two side-effects of each group?

(b) Given an example of a drug in each group.

(c) What are the contraindications of aspirin?

(d) How is paracetamol potentially lethal?

(e) What other properties does paracetamol have beside analgesia.

(f) Write a regimen for postoperative pain control for a fit and healthy patient whose lower wisdom tooth has been surgically extracted.

**Answer 7.12**

(a) Analgesics for dental pain and their side-effects:
- NSAIDs – gastric ulceration, asthma attacks
- Aspirin (can be included in NSAIDs) – gastric ulceration, asthma attacks, allergic disease, Reye syndrome, hepatic impairment
- Opioids – respiratory depression, nausea, vomiting, constipation, dependence
- Paracetamol – liver damage, rashes, blood disorders (thrombocytopenia, leucopenia)

(b) Any one of the following:
- NSAIDs – ibuprofen, ketoprofen, diclofenac, mefenamic acid
- Aspirin
- Opioids – morphine, codeine, diamorphine, dihydrocodeine, codeine phosphate, fentanyl, papaveretum,
- Paracetamol

(c) Contraindications of aspirin:
- Bleeding disorders
- Gastric or duodenal ulceration
- Patient under 12 years
- Asthma
- Pregnancy
- Allergy to aspirin

(d) It can cause liver toxicity

(e) It is antipyretic.

(f) Postoperative pain control:
- Ibuprofen – 400 mg up to four times daily orally as required
- Paracetamol – 1g up to four times daily orally as required

- Dihydrocodeine 30 mg up to four times daily orally as required
- Codeine phosphate 30mg up to four times daily orally as required

**7.13** (a) A 40-year-old woman comes to your surgery for a dental extraction. Her medical history reveals that she has had endocarditis. She is not allergic to anything that she is aware of. What precautions would you take before the extraction?

(b) After she has taken what you prescribed for her she rapidly developed swelling of her lips. What is the likely diagnosis?

- Anaphylaxis
- Angioedema
- Cheilitis granulomatous
- Orofacial granulomatosis

(c) Name four other clinical signs and symptoms that patients may have in this condition.

(d) How is this condition managed?

## Answer 7.13

(a) The patient requires antibiotic cover. Using the BNF guidelines this would involve giving the patient iv amoxicillin 1g and iv gentamycin 120mg prior to the procedure followed by 500mg amoxicillin six hours later orally. Using the BSAC guidelines this would involve giving the patient 3g oral amoxicillin one hour before the procedure.

(b) Anaphylaxis

(c) Any four of the following:
- Erythema
- Urticaria
- Wheezing
- Bronchospasm
- Hypotension
- Thready pulse

(d) Management of anaphylaxis:
- Adrenaline (epinephrine) – 0.5–1 ml of 1:1000 intramuscularly
- Hydrocortisone – 100 mg intravenously
- Chlorphenamine – 10 mg intravenously
- Oxygen inhalation

**7.14** (a) You are carrying out a dental extraction on a 70-year-old man in your practice. He pushes your hand away and tells you to stop leaning on his chest (which you are not doing). What is the likely diagnosis?

(b) What other symptoms may he be experiencing?

(c) How would you proceed in this situation?

(d) The pain continues and becomes more severe. He becomes pale, clammy and feels nauseous. What has happened?

(e) How would you proceed?

## Answer 7.14

(a) Ischaemic chest pain (angina)

(b) The patient may also be experiencing:
- Central chest /retrosternal pain
- Band-like chest pain
- Pain radiating to the mandible/left arm

(c) Management of ischaemic chest pain:
1 Stop the procedure.
2 Make the patient sit up.
3 Administer sublingual GTN.
4 Administer oxygen.

(d) The ischaemic chest pain has progressed from angina (reversible) to myocardial infarction (irreversible).

(e) Management of myocardial infarction:
1 Call for help (ambulance).
2 Continue to give oxygen.
3 Establish intravenous access (useful for analgesia (opioids) but you probably would not have these in general practice). Also helpful should patient progress to cardiac arrest.
4 Give analgesia nitrous oxide/oxygen mixture (50% oxygen).
5 Give aspirin (300 mg).

**7.15** (a) A pregnant woman needs to have dental treatment. When is the best time for carrying out the treatment and why?

(b) What are the potential problems with carrying out treatment at other times?

(c) What oral conditions may a pregnant woman present with?

(d) If a pregnant woman had a dental abscess, which of the following antibiotics can you prescribe for her?

- Penicillin

- Erythromycin

- Metronidazole

(e) If you needed to prescribe analgesics which ones could you prescribe and which ones would you avoid and why?

## Answer 7.15

(a) Ideally major dental work should be delayed until after pregnancy. The best time to carry out treatment during pregnancy is probably the second trimester as it is important not to neglect dental health, eg pregnancy periodontitis.

(b) During the first trimester the fetus is most susceptible to teratogenic influences and abortion; 15% of pregnancies terminate in the first trimester. In the third trimester the risk of syncope is highest. Pressure on the inferior vena cava when the woman is supine leads to reduced venous return and hypotension. There is also the risk of pre-eclampsia.

(c) Oral conditions in pregnancy:
- Pyogenic granuloma /epulis
- Exacerbation of pre-existing gingivitis/periodontitis
- Pregnancy periodontitis

(d) In pregnancy the following can be prescribed:
- Penicillin
- Erythromycin

Note: Drugs can have harmful effects on the fetus during pregnancy. During the first trimester there is the risk of teratogenesis (congenital malformation), and during the second and third trimesters, drugs may affect growth and functional development. Near term they may have adverse effects on labour or on the neonate after delivery.

(e) Paracetamol can be prescribed in pregnancy. It is not known to be harmful in pregnancy. Avoid opioid analgesics (eg codeine, tramadol, morphine). They can cause neonatal respiratory depression and withdrawal. NSAIDs can be associated with a risk of premature closure of the ductus arteriosus so they are contraindicated in the third trimester.

**7.16** (a) What are the three characteristic features of asthma?

(b) Give three clinical features and signs that would make you suspect asthma in a patient.

(c) Name three groups of agents that are used in the treatment of asthma. How do they work?

(d) A 20-year-old patient with known asthma and concurrent coryza comes for dental treatment. During treatment he develops chest tightening and wheezing. How would you proceed?

## Answer 7.16

(a) Characteristic features of asthma:
  - Reversible airflow limitation
  - Airway hyper-responsiveness to a range of stimuli
  - Inflammation of the bronchi

(b) Any three of the following:
  - Episodic wheeze or cough
  - Shortness of breath
  - Diurnal variation (symptoms worse at night and early morning)
  - Expiratory polyphonic wheeze on auscultation
  - Reduced chest expansion during asthma attack

(c) There is a stepwise approach in the management of a patient with asthma, which depends partly on their peak flow.
  1 $\beta_2$-adrenoreceptor agonists (eg salbutamol, terbutaline, salmeterol) – causes relaxation of bronchial smooth muscle and bronchial dilatation
  2 Anticholinergic bronchodilator (eg ipratropium bromide) – causes bronchodilatation
  3 Inhaled corticosteroids (eg beclomethasone, budesonide) – they are anti-inflammatory agents used as maintenance treatment
  4 Sodium cromoglicate – prevents activation of inflammatory cells
  5 Slow-release theophylline – relaxes smooth muscle

(d) Management of patient with known asthma and concurrent coryza:
  1 Stop treatment.
  2 Make the patient sit upright
  3 Follow ABC.
  4 Clear the patient's airway, use suction, if necessary. Remove all instruments. Check the patient has not inhaled any foreign body. If so remove or use the Heimlich manoeuvre.

**5** Give two puffs of salbutamol inhaler.

**6** Give oxygen.

**7** If patient still short of breathe give hydrocortisone 100 mg intravenously.

**8** Call for help.

**7.17** (a) Select from the list below two conditions that diabetes mellitus may be secondary to:

- Corticosteroid treatment
- Chronic pancreatitis
- Obesity
- Insulin overproduction
- Insulin insufficiency
- Insulin resistance
- Insulin sensitivity

(b) Which of the above happens with regard to insulin?

(c) List four presenting features of diabetes mellitus.

(d) What dental manifestations may a diabetic patient present with?

(e) What is the most common diabetic emergency likely to present in general dental practice? What are the symptoms of this condition?

(f) If this condition occurs how would you manage it?

**Answer 7.17**

(a) Any two of the following:
- Corticosteroid treatment
- Chronic pancreatitis
- Obesity
- Insulin insufficiency
- Insulin resistance

(b)
- Insulin insufficiency
- Insulin resistance

(c) Any four of the following:
- Polyuria
- Polydipsia
- Weight loss
- Lethargy
- Recurrent infection

(d) Oral manifestations of diabetes:
- Chronic periodontal disease
- Increased susceptibility to infections/dental abscesses
- Xerostomia

(e) Hypoglycaemia. The patient may be irritable, disorientated, increasingly drowsy, excitable or aggressive. They may appear drunk, cold, sweaty and tachycardic.

(f) Check the blood glucose level to verify hypoglycaemia if you have the facility to do so otherwise presume hypoglycaemic episode. Then:
  - If conscious give glucose orally in any form.

  - If unconscious place in recovery position, give 1 mg glucagon intramuscularly, or obtain intravenous access and administer 50 ml of 20–50% dextrose.

Note: In a diabetic patient it is safer to give glucose and not insulin if there are any concerns about the diagnosis.

**7.18** (a) A new patient attends your practice with a medical history of epilepsy. What is epilepsy?

(b) Name two common types of epilepsy.

(c) Phenytoin is often given to patients to control their epilepsy. What are the dental implications of a patient taking phenytoin?

(d) Name two other drugs that are often used to control epilepsy?

(e) What do you understand by the term status epilepticus and how would you manage it in the dental surgery?

## Answer 7.18

(a) It is a spontaneous intermittent abnormal electrical activity in a part of the brain that results in seizures.

(b) Any two of the following:
- Grand mal epilepsy
- Petit mal epilepsy
- Myoclonic
- Simple and complex focal seizures

(c) Patients given long-term phenytoin treatment may develop gingival hyperplasia.

(d) Any two of the following:
- Carbamazepine
- Sodium valproate
- Phenobarbitone
- Benzodiazepines
- Lamotrigine

(e) In status epilepticus the fitting does not stop after 15 minutes or fits are rapidly repeated without intervening consciousness. Management involves:
- 10mg intravenous diazepam over 2 minutes (0.5 mg/kg body weight can be administered by the rectal route if intravenous access is difficult, but as this is not a commonly used route for drug administration in the dental surgery do not use it unless you know what you are doing)
- Maintain airway and administer oxygen
- Call for help (ambulance)
- Repeat diazepam if no recovery after 5 minutes

**7.19** (a) What do you understand by the terms bacteraemia and septicaemia?

(b) Infective endocarditis may occur as a complication of dental treatment – what is infective endocarditis?

(c) Which organisms commonly cause infective endocarditis?

(d) Which patients are at risk of getting infective endocarditis from dental treatment?

(e) What precautions should be taken before carrying out subgingival scaling under local anaesthetic in a patient who has had previous endocarditis if they are allergic to penicillin?

## Answer 7.19

(a) Bacteraemia means bacteria in the blood stream, usually at a low level and clinically not of consequence. Septicaemia is sepsis in the blood stream and is due to large numbers of organisms in the blood. Clinical features include rigours, fever and hypotension.

(b) Inflammation of the endocardium of the heart valves and endocardium around congenital defects of the heart from an infection.

(c) Bacteria most commonly cause infective endocarditis – usually *Streptococcus viridans*, *Streptococcus faecalis* (subacute infective endocarditis) and *Streptococcus pneumoniae*, *Staphylococcus aureus* and *Streptococcus pyogenes* (acute infective endocarditis); fungi, chlamydia and rickettsiae less commonly cause this condition.

(d) Those who have had previous endocarditis, those with prosthetic heart valves and those with surgically constructed systemic or pulmonary shunts or conduits. (Note: This is following the British Society for Antimicrobial Chemotherapy 2006 guidelines).

(e) Give 600 mg oral clindamycin 1 hour preoperatively.

**7.20** (a) A 40-year-old man presents with a medical history of alcoholic liver disease and needs a dental extraction. What are your concerns and why?

(b) He is very anxious and requests sedation. Are there any contraindications?

(c) Which antibiotic could you safely prescribe this patient from the list below:

- Amoxicillin
- Flucloxacillin
- Erythromycin
- Tetracycline
- Doxycycline
- Metronidazole
- Clindamycin
- Cephalosporins

(d) The following is a list of commonly used drugs in dentistry. If you had a patient with renal failure how would this affect the prescription of the drugs? For each drug state whether you would prescribe it normally, reduce the dose or avoid it completely

- Amoxicillin
- Metronidazole
- Tetracycline
- Miconazole
- Midazolam
- NSAIDs

## Answer 7.20

(a) Alcoholic liver disease is a cause of liver cirrhosis. The liver is responsible for plasma proteins including clotting factors and for detoxification. The patient may have excessive bleeding following the extraction, so it is important to check for a history of abnormal bleeding.

(b) Due to reduced drug clearance, the use of sedatives should be avoided as coma is a risk.

(c) Amoxicillin, flucloxacillin, cephalosporins

(d) Dose alterations in renal failure:
  - Amoxicillin – reduce dose
  - Metronidazole – prescribe normally
  - Tetracycline – avoid
  - Miconazole – reduce dose
  - Midazolam – reduce dose
  - NSAIDs – avoid

**7.21**  Look at the full blood count (FBC) results and choose from the list below the condition the patient may have, the appearance on the blood film and the possible causes.

- Macrocytic anaemia
- Microcytic anaemia
- Hypochromic anaemia
- Normocytic anaemia
- Iron deficiency
- $B_{12}$ deficiency
- Folate deficiency
- Anaemia of chronic disease
- Thalassaemia
- Blood loss
- Alcoholism

(a) Full blood count:

| | | Reference interval |
|---|---|---|
| Haemoglobin (Hb) | 108 g/l | 135–180 g/l (female), 115–160 g/l (male) |
| Packed cell volume (PCV) | 0.33 l/l | 0.37–0.47 l/l (female), 0.4–0.54 l/l (male) |
| Mean corpuscular volume (MCV) | 72 fl | 76–79 fl |
| Mean corpuscular haemoglobin (MCH) | 25 pg | 27–32 pg |
| Mean corpuscular haemoglobin concentration (MCHC) | 280 g/l | 300–360 g/l |
| White cell count (WCC) | $6.6 \times 10^9$/l | $4.0–11 \times 10^9$/l |
| Platelets | $207 \times 10^9$/l | $150–400 \times 10^9$/l |

(b) Full blood count:

| | | Reference interval |
|---|---|---|
| Haemoglobin (Hb) | 98 g/l | 135–180 g/l (female), 115–160 g/l (male) |
| Packed cell volume (PCV) | 0.6 l/l | 0.37–0.47 l/l (female), 0.4–0.54 l/l (male) |
| Mean corpuscular volume (MCV) | 84 fl | 76–79 fl |
| Mean corpuscular haemoglobin (MCH) | 28 pg | 27–32 pg |
| Mean corpuscular haemoglobin concentration (MCHC) | 320 g/l | 300–360 g/l |
| White cell count (WCC) | $8.2 \times 10^9$/l | $4.0–11 \times 10^9$/l |
| Platelets | $255 \times 10^9$/l | $150–400 \times 10^9$/l |

(c) List five signs and symptoms of anaemia (not including intraoral ones).

## Answer 7.21

(a) FBC shows microcytic hypochromic anaemia:
- Microcytic anaemia
- Hypochromic anaemia
- Iron deficiency
- Thalassaemia
- Blood loss

(b) FBC shows macrocytic anaemia consistent with:
- $B_{12}$ deficiency
- Folate deficiency
- Alcoholism

(b) The signs depend on the severity of the anaemia. They range from lethargy, pallor and weakness to dizziness, tinnitus, vertigo, headache and dyspnoea (shortness of breath) on exertion, tachycardia, palpitations, angina, cardiac failure and gastrointestinal disturbances.

**7.22** Give two features seen in each of the syndromes listed below.

| Syndrome | Features |
|---|---|
| Apert | |
| Crouzon | |
| Treacher Collins | |
| Albright | |
| Pierre–Robin | |
| Goldenhar | |
| Van der Woude | |
| Gardener | |
| Down | |
| Gorlin–Goltz | |
| Ramsay–Hunt | |
| Peutz–Jeghers | |

## Answer 7.22

Any two of the features given in the table below:

| Syndrome | Features |
| --- | --- |
| Apert | Craniosynostosis (premature closure of sutures of skull), fused fingers and toes, can be associated with cleft palate, maxillary hypoplasia |
| Crouzon | Shallow orbits, proptosis, conductive hearing loss, may have small maxilla |
| Treacher Collins | Underdeveloped or absent cheekbone and abnormal shape of the eyes, malformed or absent ears, micrognathia |
| Albright | Café-au-lait patches, polyostotic fibrous dysplasia, endocrine dysfunction, precocious puberty |
| Pierre–Robin | Prominent tongue, micrognathia, cleft palate |
| Goldenhar | Bilateral craniofacial microsomia, epibulbar dermoids, vertebral anomalies |
| Van der Woude | Lower lip pits, cleft lip |
| Gardener | Multiple osteomas, intestinal polyps, cysts, skin fibromas |
| Down | Flattened nasal bridge, upward sloping palpebral fissures, midface retrusion, Class III malocclusion, macroglossia, delayed tooth eruption, heart defects, atlantoaxial subluxation |
| Gorlin–Goltz | Basal cell carcinomas, keratocysts, parietal bossing, bifid ribs, calcification of the falx cerebri |
| Ramsay–Hunt | Lower motor neurone facial palsy, vesicles, herpes zoster of the geniculate ganglion |
| Peutz–Jeghers | Intestinal polyps, perioral pigmentation |

**7.23** (a) A new patient has collapsed in your waiting room. Outline your initial management of the situation.

(b) If he is unresponsive how will you proceed?

(c) If you need to do cardiopulmonary resuscitation what ratio of chest compressions to breaths will you use?

(d) How many chest compressions are you aiming to complete per minute?

(e) Where will you place your hands to do the compressions?

(f) By how much are you attempting to compress the chest?

(g) How long should you take over your rescue breaths?

(i) How long are you going to continue resuscitating for?

## Answer 7.23

(a) Initial management:
   1 Check the area is safe.

   2 Try to arouse the patient by shaking and shouting to him in both ears.

   3 If there is no response shout for help and proceed to resuscitation.

(b) If the patient is unresponsive:
   1 Shout for help.

   2 Follow ABC resuscitation guidelines.

   3 Check airway and clear it and open it if necessary.

   4 Check breathing – look, listen and feel for no more than 10 seconds.

   5 If there are no signs of breathing go for help and call ambulance (or get someone else to go if you are not alone).

   6 Give 30 chest compressions.

   7 Give 2 rescue breaths.

   8 Give 30 chest compressions, etc.

(c) 30 compressions to 2 breaths

(d) 100

(e) In the centre of the chest

(f) About 4 cm in an adult per compression

(g) 1 second for each breath

(i) Until help comes or you become exhausted or the patient recovers (Note: This is based on the Resuscitation Council UK Guidelines 2005)

**7.24** The following are drugs that you may have in your emergency box. In which conditions and how you would use them? How you would recognise each condition?

- Glyceryl trinitrate

- Adrenaline

- Salbutamol

- Aspirin

## Answer 7.24

- Glyceryl trinitrate – sublingual spray or tablet, used in angina. Angina is acute chest pain due to myocardial ischaemia. Patients feel central crushing chest pain which may radiate down their left arm or a band like chest pain. There may also be shortness of breath.

- Adrenaline – intramuscularly 0.5–1 ml of 1:1000. Given in anaphylaxis, which usually occurs following administration of a drug. Patients have facial flushing with itching or tingling. There may be facial oedema and lip swelling and urticaria. There is bronchospasm (wheezing) and hypotension. If not treated there will be loss of consciousness and cardiac arrest.

- Salbutamol – two puffs from inhaler in asthma. If there is no response use a salbutamol nebuliser. Asthmatic patients experience breathlessness, wheeze on expiration and inability to talk. They will use their accessory muscles of respiration in an attempt to breathe. Tachycardia and cyanosis may also occur.

- Aspirin – 300 mg oral in myocardial infarction. Patients have a central crushing chest pain, which does not respond to glyceryl trinitrate. There may be vomiting, sweating, pallor, cold clammy skin and shortness of breathe and the patient may progress to loss of consciousness.

**7.25** (a) What is shock?

(b) Septic and cardiogenic are two different types of shock. Name two other types of shock.

(c) Fill in the blanks in the table about the features of a particular type of shock.

| Type of shock | Associated features | Peripheral temperature | Central venous pressure |
|---|---|---|---|
|  | Dehydrated/ blood loss |  | Reduced |

Note: Peripheral temperature may be increased, decreased or stay the same.

(d) What do you understand by the term Addisonian crisis?

(e) If this occurs in the dental surgery how should it be managed?

## Answer 7.25

(a) Shock is acute circulatory failure leading to inadequate tissue perfusion and end organ injury or inadequate tissue oxygenation/organ perfusion.

(b) Any two of the following:
  • Hypovolaemic
  • Anaphylactic
  • Neurogenic

(c)

| Type of shock | Associated features | Peripheral temperature | Central venous pressure |
|---------------|---------------------|------------------------|-------------------------|
| Hypovolaemic | Dehydrated/ blood loss | Decreased | Reduced |

(d) In Addison's disease there is a failure of secretion of cortisol and aldosterone and patients are treated with steroids. In times of stress such as infections, surgery or anaesthesia the body cannot respond due to the inadequate corticosteroid production. This results in a rapid fall in blood pressure, which leads to circulatory collapse and shock. This is known as Addisonian crisis.

(e) Management of Addisonian crisis:
  1 Lie the patient flat and raise their legs.
  2 Give hydrocortisone sodium succinate 100–200 mg intravenously.
  3 Call for help (ambulance).
  4 Oxygen.
  5 IV fluids may be administered but only if you are familiar with their use.

# 8
# General Dentistry

**8.1**   What do the following commonly used abbreviations stand for?

- IOTN
- OM radiograph
- BPE
- dmfs
- DMFS
- INR
- ESR
- CPITN
- MMPA
- MTA

## Answer 8.1

- IOTN – Index of Treatment Need
- OM radiograph – occipitomental radiograph
- BPE – Basic Periodontal Examination
- dmfs – decayed missing and filled tooth surfaces of deciduous teeth
- DMFT – decayed missing and filled teeth in permanent teeth
- INR – international normalised ratio (used for measuring the efficacy of and monitoring anticoagulant treatment)
- ESR – erythrocyte sedimentation rate
- CPITN – Community Periodontal Index of Treatment Need
- MMPA – maxillary–mandibular planes angle
- MTA – mineral trioxide aggregate

**8.2**  (a) Dental practices should have a written infection control protocol. List six elements that should be included in this document?

(b) How can clinical staff protect themselves from the risk of infection from patients?

(c) What do you understand by the term universal precautions?

(d) Name one condition for which additional measures are used.

## Answer 8.2

(a) Any six of the following:
- Patient evaluation
- Personal protection
- Staff training in infection control measures
- Instrument management with respect to cleaning, sterilisation and storage
- Disinfection
- Disposable instruments
- Waste disposal
- Laboratory asepsis

(b) Protection against cross-infection (patient to staff):
- Immunisation against certain infectious diseases, eg hepatitis B, rubella, tuberculosis
- Wearing gloves
- Wearing eye protection glasses/visors/goggles
- Wearing appropriate clothing
- Handwashing
- Reducing aerosols in the surgery by using high-volume aspirators
- Using rubber dam for restorative procedures where appropriate
- Not re-sheathing needles

(c) This term means that all patients are treated equally with regards to cross-infection control, as normal measures should be of such a standard to prevent cross-infection. In other words, every patient is treated as though they were potentially infectious.

(d) Transmissible spongiform encephalopathy/Creutzfeldt–Jacob disease/new variant Creutzfeldt–Jacob disease

**8.3** (a) Many instruments are sterilised in autoclaves, how does this differ from a hot air oven and what are the advantages of using an autoclave?

(b) Give one example regimen of how an autoclave achieves sterilisation?

(c) What methods are used to test that an autoclave is working effectively?

**Answer 8.3**

(a) Hot air ovens use dry heat to kill micro-organisms and spores. They usually achieve temperatures of 160–180 °C, but at least an hour at this temperature is required for the procedure to be effective. Autoclaves use moist heat under pressure for sterilisation, this allows higher temperatures to be reached and so reduces the sterilisation time. Steam also contracts in volume during condensation, which increases penetration as well as liberates latent heat. Both these increase microbicidal activity.

(b) Any one of the following:
- 121–124 °C for 15 minutes at 104 kPa

- 134–137 °C for 3 minutes at 207 kPa

(c) Methods for testing autoclaves:
- Mechanical indicators on machine, eg temperature and pressure dials will tell you when appropriate settings have been reached.

- Process indicators are paper strips or liquids that change colour when they have been exposed to the appropriate settings. They will not prove that there are no pathogens remaining, just that the appropriate conditions were reached.

- Biological indicators actually prove that sterilisation has occurred. They contain bacterial spores which will lose their viability if the appropriate cycle conditions are reached. The indicators are removed from the autoclave and are cultured. If the spores are viable then the autoclave is not achieving sterilisation.

**8.4** (a) What is the difference between sterilisation and disinfection?

(b) Name two items in a dental environment that are disinfected rather than sterilised.

(c) Chemicals are often used for disinfection. Name one other method of disinfection used in dentistry

(d) Name three chemicals that may be used for disinfection in dentistry.

(e) What do you understand by the term antisepsis and when would it be used?

## Answer 8.4

(a) Sterilisation is the removal of all living micro-organisms and their pathogenic products whereas disinfection removes some of the micro-organisms, usually the pathogenic ones.

(b) Any two of the following:
- Work surfaces in the surgery
- Light handles, chair arms, headrest, spittoon, etc.
- Patient safety glasses
- Impressions
- Collimating device

(c) Any one of the following:
- Heat (eg boiling)
- Physical (eg ultrasonics)

(d) Any three of the following:
- Alcohols
- Biguanides (eg chlorhexidine)
- Glutaraldehyde (this is banned in some areas)
- Chlorines
- Phenols

(e) Antisepsis is the application of a chemical agent externally on a live surface (eg skin or mucosa) to destroy organisms or to inhibit their growth. For example, preparing the skin prior to an operation or prior to taking a blood sample.

**8.5** (a) What treatment should dirty but re-usable dental instruments undergo prior to sterilisation and why?

(b) How is this carried out?

(c) If items are not re-usable, they need to be disposed. How do you dispose the following items?

- Suture needle

- Blood-stained gauze

- Waste amalgam

- Old record cards

(d) What do you understand by the term 'clinical waste'?

**Answer 8.5**

(a) All dirty instruments need to be cleaned prior to sterilisation to remove debris and organic material. This is because organic material (eg saliva and blood) remaining on instruments will increase the chances of survival of bacteria and can interfere with the sterilisation process. This cleaning process may be called pre-sterilisation or decontamination.

(b) Instruments can be scrubbed manually or cleaned in an ultrasonic bath.

(c) Methods of appropriate disposal:
   - Suture needle – into a rigid sharps bin that will be incinerated.

   - Blood-stained gauze – in a clinical waste bag (usually yellow bag) that will be incinerated.

   - Amalgam – waste amalgam should be stored under liquid in a closed container until such time as it is collected by a specialised amalgam waste disposal service for disposal. It must not be put into clinical waste for incineration as mercury vapour will be produced.

   - Old record cards – these contain confidential patient information so must not just be put in domestic waste. They must be disposed in such a way that patient information may not be read (by shredding or burning).

(d) Clinical waste is any waste that may be hazardous to any person coming into contact with it due to contamination with body fluids, eg blood and saliva.

**8.6** (a) Clinical records are essential to the delivery of healthcare. What are such records?

(b) Give four examples of items used in dental treatment that would be classified as 'records'.

(c) Who has access to clinical records?

(d) For how long should dental records be kept?

(e) Computerised and manual patient records in dental practice are governed by which law in the UK and when was it introduced?

(f) Give three statements from this law.

## Answer 8.6

(a) A medical record is any record which contains information relating to the physical or mental health or condition of an individual and has been made by or on behalf of a medical professional in connection with treatment of that individual.

(This definition is taken from the Health Professions Council.)

(b) Any four of the following:
- Clinical notes, whether handwritten or computerised
- Radiographs or other imaging records
- Photographs
- Study models
- Reports of investigations (eg laboratory reports)
- Correspondence about the patient
- Any recordings of the patient or conversations about the patient

(c) People who can access clinical records:
- Healthcare professionals involved in treating the patient
- The patient
- An insurance company paying for the treatment
- A court or the police (only when needed for investigation in a particular crime)

Note: Confidential information may be shared if it is in the public interest, but you must be able to justify your decision.

(d) Length of time records should be kept:
- For adults – 11 years after the conclusion of treatment.
- For minors – until the age of 25 or 11 years since the conclusion of treatment, whichever is longer.

Note: This is not law but is what the defence organisations suggest as good practice.

(e) 1988 Data Protection Act

(f) Any three of the following:
- Data must be held securely.
- Data must be obtained fairly and for a specific and lawful purpose.
- Data must be used only for specific and lawful purposes.
- The patient should be able to access their data if they request it.
- Data should be adequate and relevant and not be excessive.
- Data should be disclosed only to certain individuals.

**8.7** (a) Patients need to give consent for dental treatment. List five conditions that must be fulfilled for consent to be described as informed when treating an adult.

(b) What types of informed consent are there? Explain what they are.

(c) For which types of treatment is consent needed?

(d) When must a patient sign a consent form?

**Answer 8.7**

(a) Five conditions that must be fulfilled for consent:
- Patient aged over 16 years (unless they are Gillick/Fraser competent).
- Consent must be freely given.
- All risks and benefits must be explained to patient and the patient must understand them.
- All treatment options must be given to the patient.
- The patient must be able to understand and give consent (ie competent).

(b) Types of consent:
- Implied consent – the patient's actions imply that they are happy for the treatment to commence. For example a patient sitting in the dental chair and opening their mouth for an examination.
- Verbal consent – the treatment is explained to the patient and the patient agrees verbally to it.
- Written consent – the patient signs a form to say that they agree to the treatment being carried out. It is usually reserved for conditions when the patient's level of consciousness will be altered and they do not have the capacity to terminate the treatment if they wanted to.

(c) All types of treatment require consent, otherwise it is classified as assault.

(d) Procedures in which consciousness is altered – intravenous sedation and general anaesthesia. It is also useful to ask patients to sign a consent form when there is a risk of serious complications, eg damage to the inferior dental or lingual nerve during surgical removal of lower third molars.

**8.8**  (a) What does the abbreviation GDC stand for and what is the principal role of this body?

(b) What are the statutory responsibilities of the GDC?

(c) How much time for continuing professional development is required by the GDC over a period of 5 years, and into what categories is it divided?

(d) Who must be registered with the GDC?

## Answer 8.8

(a) General Dental Council. The GDC is the regulatory body of the dental profession and professions complementary to dentistry. The principal role is protecting the public.

(b) Statutory responsibilities of the GDC:
   - To promote, at all stages, high standards of education in all aspects of dentistry.

   - To promote high standards of professional conduct, performance and practice among persons registered under The Dentist Act 1984.

(c) In a 5-year cycle 250 hours of CPD must be carried out of which 75 must be verifiable. In the verifiable CPD time, 10 hours must be dedicated to medical emergencies, 5 hours to disinfection and decontamination and 5 hours to radiography and radiation protection.

(d) All dentists, dental hygienists and therapists must be registered with the GDC. Since July 2006 dental nurses and dental technicians can register; by July 2008 all must be registered with the GDC. Also no-one can call themselves a clinical dental technician or an orthodontic therapist unless they are registered with the GDC.

**8.9** (a) What do you understand by the term 'dental negligence'?

(b) Claims of negligence have to be made within certain time limits. What are these limits?

(c) Patients have the right to complain about aspects of their treatment. If a patient wishes to complain about treatment in a dental practice how should the process be conducted?

**Answer 8.9**

(a) This term means the dentist had a duty of care that was breached and that damage resulted from that breach of care.

(b) Within 3 years from the date of the knowledge of the negligence occurring or 6 years from the incident occurring or within 6 years of reaching the age of majority if the negligence occurred in a minor.

(c) Complaints procedure:

1    A copy of the written complaints procedure must be available for patients and a copy should be given to the patient when you acknowledge their complaint.

2    Send an acknowledgement of complaint within 3 working days.

3    Contact your dental defence organisation.

4    Respond in writing or by telephone as soon as possible, but no later than 10 working days.

5    If more time is needed to investigate the complaint you should inform the patient of this in your acknowledgment.

6    Regularly update your patient with your progress in investigating the complaint, at least every 10 working days.

7    Offer an apology and practical solution.

8    If the patient is not satisfied tell them about the NHS complaints procedures (or the Dental Complaints Service for private patients).

9    Patients have the right to appeal to their primary care trust for an independent review panel, or to the Healthcare Commission, and if not satisfied they can approach the NHS Ombudsman.

**8.10** (a) What do you understand by the term 'clinical audit'?

(b) What are the stages of an audit cycle?

(c) Dental professionals have a duty of care to their patients and must put patient's interests first. In what circumstances would you have a responsibility to raise any concern you have that patients might be at risk?

**Answer 8.10**

(a) This is the systematic critical analysis of the quality of clinical care, including procedures used for diagnosis and treatment, use of resources and patient outcome.

(b) Stages of an audit cycle:

    **1**  Identify the procedure or treatment method that is to be audited.

    **2**  Set the standards.

    **3**  Measure the performance against the standard that you have set.

    **4**  Analyse the results. If the standard has not been reached then clarify the problem and determine what changes need to be introduced to achieve the standard.

    **5**  Implement change.

    **6**  Re-measure the performance following implementation against the standard.

(c) If you believed patients might be at risk because:

- Of the health, behaviour or professional performance of a colleague or employer.

- Of any aspect of the clinical environment.

- Or if you have been asked to carry out any action that you believe conflicts with your duty to put patients' interests first.

**8.11**   You are suturing an extraction socket and you accidentally prick
yourself with the suture needle (needlestick injury). How should you
now proceed?

## Answer 8.11

1   Stop what you are doing.

2   Encourage the wound to bleed.

3   Wash it under running water and use a detergent if available but do not scrub.

4   Cover with waterproof plaster.

5   A risk assessment of the patient needs to be carried out – this is usually done by another person so as to eliminate a conflict of interest. The status of the patient with respect to transmissible diseases needs to be assessed; usually the patient is tested for hepatitis B and C and human immunodeficiency virus (HIV) after the risk assessment.

6   Your hepatitis B status should be assessed. As the needle is not a hollow bore needle and you would have been wearing gloves the risk is lower.

7   The incident should be recorded in an incident book.

8   Ensure that the patient's treatment is completed.

9   If there is any cause for concern you should liaise with your local point of contact for accidental body fluid exposures. This may be your occupational health department/accident and emergency department/ microbiologist/physician, depending on where you work.

Note: Local policies may differ slightly.

**8.12** (a) What does IR(ME)R stand for, and when did these regulations come into force.

(b) According to IR(ME)R what is the role of the following people and who may undertake these roles?

(i) Referrer

(ii) Practitioner

(iii) Operator

(iv) Employer

**Answer 8.12**

(a) IR(ME)R stands for Ionising Radiation (Medical Exposure) Regulations and they came into force in 2000.

(b) Description of the roles:

(i) A referrer is responsible for supplying the practitioner with sufficient information to justify the radiograph being taken. They are usually a dentist or doctor but other healthcare professionals with appropriate training may be entitled to refer patients for radiographs.

(ii) A practitioner justifies that the radiograph is necessary and that the benefits outweigh the risks. They are usually a dentist or doctor although other healthcare professionals who are entitled to take responsibility may assume the role of practitioner.

(iii) An operator is any person who carries out part or all of the tasks associated with taking the radiograph including actually taking the radiograph. They must be adequately trained and are usually dentists or dental nurses, hygienists and therapists who have undergone adequate training.

(iv) An employer or legal person is the person with legal responsibility for a radiological installation. They must ensure that the regulations are enforced and that good practice is followed. They are usually the practice owner.

# Index